Rowing the Eternal Sea

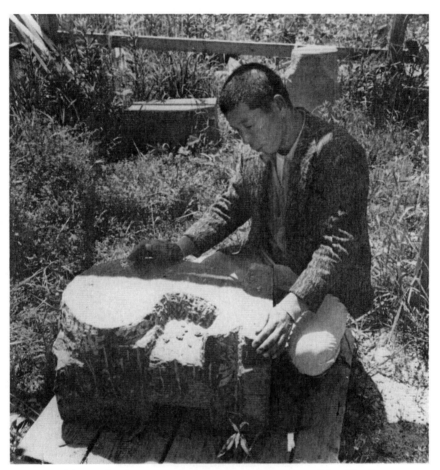

Masato planning a statue in the work area facing the reclaimed land

Rowing the Eternal Sea

The Story of a Minamata Fisherman

By Oiwa Keibo

Narrated by Ogata Masato

Translated by Karen Colligan-Taylor

ROWMAN & LITTLEFIELD PUBLISHERS, INC.
Lanham • Boulder • New York • Toronto • Plymouth, UK

ROWMAN & LITTLEFIELD PUBLISHERS, INC.

Published in the United States of America
by Rowman & Littlefield Publishers, Inc.
A wholly owned subsidiary of The Rowman & Littlefield Publishing Group, Inc.
4501 Forbes Boulevard, Suite 200, Lanham, Maryland 20706
www.rowmanlittlefield.com

10 Thornbury Road
Plymouth PL6 7PP
United Kingdom

British Library Cataloguing in Publication Information Available

Library of Congress Cataloging-in-Publication Data
Oiwa, Keibo.
  [Tokoyo no fune o kogite. English]
  Rowing the eternal sea : the story of a Minamata fisherman / by Keibo Oiwa ;
narrated by Masato Ogata ; translated by Karen Colligan-Taylor.
    p. cm. — (Asian voices)
  Includes bibliographical references and index.
  ISBN 0-7425-0020-9 (cloth : alk. paper) — ISBN 0-7425-0021-7 (pbk. : alk. paper)
    1. Mercury—Toxicology. 2. Water—Pollution—Japan—Minamata-shi. 3.
Mercury—Environmental aspects—Japan—Minamata-shi. I. Ogata, Masato, 1953–
II. Colligan-Taylor, Karen. III. Title. IV. Series.
  RA1231.M5 .O504 2001
  615.9′25663—dc21   2001040427

Printed in the United States of America

♾ ™ The paper used in this publication meets the minimum requirements of American
National Standard for Information Sciences—Permanence of Paper for Printed Library
Materials, ANSI/NISO Z39.48–1992.

We dedicate this book to the fond memory of our common friend, Higa Yasuo (1938–2000), a great photographer, ethnologist, and philosopher, who helped us see the invisible.

Oiwa Keibo and Ogata Masato

Contents

Acknowledgments   ix

Translator's Introduction   1
  Karen Colligan-Taylor

Prologue: "Out to the Mythological Sea"   17
  Ishimure Michiko

Part I
  A Vibrant Village   25
  The Bitter Sea   29
  Competing Souls   33
  What's Going On?   39
  Two Hints   43
  Within the Circle   49
  School Days   53
  A Family Ordeal   57
  Leaving Home   61
  A Compass Restored   67

Part II
  Rising Tides   73
  Social Activism   79
  Life Changes   87
  Leaving the Movement   91
  The Depths of Despair   95
  Facing My Demons   99

Tokoyo no fune, Boat to the Eternal World   103
Bearing Witness   109
A Will of Stone   117
A Place of Atonement   121

Part III
Beneath the Light of the Sun and the Moon   129
The Chisso within Us   143
Keep the Embers Glowing   151
Nusari, Embracing Life as a Gift   159
Moyainaoshi, Moored Together Again   165

Epilogue   177
  Oiwa Keibo

Index   187

About . . .
  The Author   193
  The Narrator   193
  The Translator   193

Acknowledgments

I would like to express my special gratitude to Karen Colligan-Taylor, who firmly believed in the significance of this project and worked diligently to offer a superb translation, and to Mark Selden, who patiently guided me along the long, winding path since the very beginning of this project. I am convinced that Karen and Mark are the best collaborators that I could possibly have found for this project. It has been my honor and pleasure to work with Susan McEachern of Rowman & Littlefield, our publisher; Ishimure Michiko, who generously offered the beautiful prologue; and Ogata Sawako, who made me feel at home on my numerous visits to Minamata. Photojournalists Akutagawa Jin and Shiota Takeshi, and the Soshisha Minamata Disease Center kindly contributed their photographs to this book.

I am deeply grateful for the indispensable help and guidance of the following individuals: Nina Kahori Fallenbaum, Thom Richardson, David Suzuki, Nakamura Ryuichi, Anja Light, Ogata Magumu, Yanagimoto Mari, Fujimoto Susumu, Fujimoto Akiko, Kurihara Akira, Kyoko Selden, Baco Ohama, Brenda Andrews, Loretta Todd, and Ori Arisa.

I am fortunate to be a member of the faculty of International Studies at Meiji Gakuin University, which has always been supportive of my research projects.

Finally, I thank Ogata Masato for being my friend and for being the human being that he is.

Rowing the Eternal Sea is a revision and update of *Tokoyo no fune o kogite*, by Ogata Masato and Tsuji Shin'ichi (pen name of Oiwa Keibo) (Yokohama: Seori Shobo, 1996). This is Ogata Masato's story as told to Oiwa Keibo over a period of several years. Oiwa Keibo edited and structured transcriptions of taped interviews; Ogata Masato commented on and approved the final narrative form.

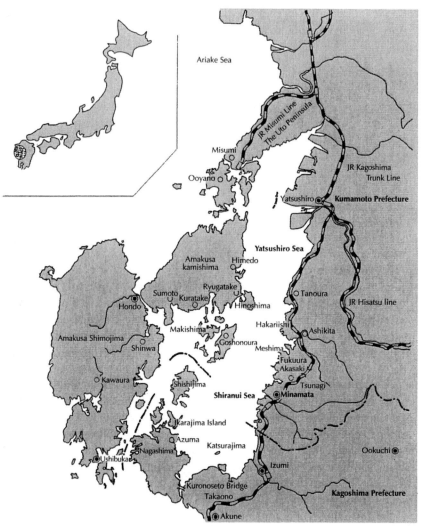

The Shiranui Sea: an inland sea bordered by Kyushu and the Amakusa Islands. Minamata is located on the ragged southern coast of the Shiranui Sea, where the many inlets and coves provide suitable spawning grounds for fish and shellfish.

Translator's Introduction

Karen Colligan-Taylor

It was in 1953 that villagers in fishing hamlets near Minamata City, on the west coast of Kyushu, Japan, first noticed their cats dancing madly. How could they know that this bizarre performance was the prelude to an environmental disaster that would grow to stigmatize their region and define their lives? That same year Ogata Masato was born to a hard-working family that made its living from the rich waters around Minamata Bay. Unaware of the disease that would soon strike the family, none of its members would have dreamed that the fish that sustained them would bring debilitation and death. For thirty-six years, from 1932 to 1968, Chisso Corporation, in the vanguard of Japan's chemical industry, used mercuric sulfate as a catalyst in the production of acetaldehyde, releasing methyl mercury in its untreated effluent. Entering the marine ecosystem, mercury was taken up in the food chain, its concentration greatly magnified at each higher level, first in plankton and sea-bottom organisms, then in fish, and finally in cats, birds, and humans.

In *Rowing the Eternal Sea*, Masato offers a personal history of Minamata disease—methyl mercury poisoning—as he describes the impact of industrial pollution on his own life, his extended family, and the fishing culture of the Shiranui Sea.[1] However, his story is bigger than one man or one incident, and it raises questions we would do well to consider as benefactors of modern industry and technology.

"Think about the difference between *kiroku* (a record, document) and *kioku* (memory)," said Masato, speaking earnestly as he drove. The narrow winding highway skirted the sea for fifteen miles from Minamata to Masato's home in Kochidomari, a fishing hamlet of eleven households in the village of Meshima. "Once you record an event *(kiroku shiteshimau)*, both the event and the act of documentation are considered complete and final, a part of the

1

past. But *kioku*, remembrance, is a living process. Culture, customs, regional history, and family stories are carried forward, from one generation to the next. In today's information society, *kiroku* (written documentation) has become an important commodity. But the way I want to communicate the past and the way I would like everyone to remember it is through *kioku*. The Minamata incident must never be filed or shelved. It must remain alive in our collective memories."[2]

The Minamata tragedy began, Masato suggests, "when people stopped seeing their fellow humans as human beings." The episode mirrors the society that produced it. National policy drove Chisso's corporate philosophy and growth. In 1908, Chisso's parent company, Nippon Chisso Hiryo (Japan Nitrogen Fertilizer), was established in a merger of Nippon Carbide and Sogi Electric in a fishing hamlet at the mouth of the Minamata River. Local leaders welcomed this new enterprise as a replacement for the region's principal cash-earning industries, salt production—which had just been declared a government monopoly—and the transport of coal to regional mines, now supplied with hydroelectric power. In this poor, seaside district Chisso proceeded to build a "castle town," which attracted labor and service industries from outlying districts.[3] Tracks were laid to Minamata, and a train station was built at Chisso's front gate. A nearby village, Umedo, became a thriving port. The population grew steadily. As the leading industrial firm in Kumamoto Prefecture, Chisso easily dominated regional politics, channeling municipal funds into "public" works designed specifically to promote factory expansion. The company played the role of the beneficent overlord, never allowing local residents to forget that "Minamata exists at the grace of Chisso."[4]

Although Japan began a rapid program of modernization in 1868, social attitudes changed slowly. "Peasants are like sesame seeds," went a popular saying of the feudal period. "The more you squeeze, the more they produce." Japan's early twentieth-century labor force fared no better. Chisso's founder, Noguchi Shitagau, is famous for his alleged directive, "*Shokko o ningen toshite tsukauna, gyuba to omotte tsukae* (Don't treat the workers as humans; think of them as cows and horses)."[5] In 1927 Chisso built another industrial complex in colonial Korea, based on large-scale hydroelectric power generation. Hungnam (Konan), a fishing village of three thousand, soon boasted a population of two hundred thousand. Compared with their Japanese counterparts, Korean workers hired at the plant received significantly lower wages and inferior housing. The Japanese army backed Chisso's overseas operation, ensuring that laborers accepted their lot.[6]

In the 1920s Chisso produced fertilizers, synthetic fibers, explosives, oils, and industrial chemicals. Expanding its operations in Minamata, Chisso received a patent for the synthesis of acetic acid in 1931 and began operation of an acetaldehyde plant in 1932, making use of new technology employing mercuric sulphate. The production of vinyl chloride, also catalyzed by mercury, began in 1941.[7] Untreated wastewater laden with heavy metals was discharged directly into Minamata Bay at Hyakken Port. Even before the discharge of mercury, however, pollution incidents had affected the local fishery. The earliest compensation payments by Chisso to fishing cooperatives for a fishery decline date from 1926.[8]

Occupational hazards inside the plant were as appalling as environmental pollution outside. From the 1930s, workers in experimental pilot plants reported acid burns and death or injury from frequent explosions.[9] While white-collar workers at the company received high salaries with many perks, blue-collar workers earned relatively low salaries and were considered expendable commodities in the production process. Nonetheless, laborers enjoyed higher status than fishermen and farmers, whom they shunned as the lowest of the low.

Following Japan's defeat in World War II, Chisso was stripped of its overseas assets, leaving it with only the Minamata factory complex. Due to the effects of the war Japan's chemical industry was slow to recover, but by rebuilding its hydroelectric plant, Chisso was soon back in production. A visit from Emperor Hirohito in 1949 underlined Chisso's importance in the postwar economy.[10] At this time there was a great demand for polyvinyl chloride (PVC), and Chisso had a monopoly on the production of octanol, a derivative of acetaldehyde and a key ingredient in plastics.

Continuing to rely on electrochemical technology, however, Chisso missed out on the first wave of technological innovation from electro- to petrochemistry; it hastened to catch up by joining with Maruzen Sekiyu Corporation in the mid 1950s to establish a petrochemical factory in the town of Goi, Chiba Prefecture. In order to fund the Goi venture, Chisso's Minamata factory was required to work at full capacity using outdated equipment. Only in 1966, when the new petrochemistry plant was completed in Goi, did the Ministry of International Trade and Industry (MITI) encourage Chisso to modernize its Minamata facility.[11] Large amounts of mercury compounds continued to be used as production catalysts, and wastewater was discharged without treatment. Concerns for human and environmental health did not enter the national policy-making process, which had long sacrificed rural society and ecosystems for urban prosperity.

In the decade 1955 to 1965, the period of greatest outbreak of Minamata disease, two hundred thousand people lived along the Shiranui coast. One hundred thousand lived in the most highly affected areas.[12] Because people were affected by methyl mercury to different degrees, depending on age and extent of exposure, and because certain medical conditions worsened over time, it is impossible to identify the exact number poisoned. As of April 2001 nineteen thousand sufferers had applied for certification as Minamata disease patients.[13] But many, including Masato's father, died before the certification process was instituted and many more kept silent. Afflicted families were ostracized by relatives and neighbors. Community ties and a way of life were destroyed, leaving no one along the Shiranui coast untouched. Some of the earliest victims were identified years later through examination of organs preserved during autopsies.

One of the victims was an uncle of Masato's close friend and mentor, Kawamoto Teruo (1931–1999). Kawamoto's uncle, a professional fisherman, showed symptoms of acute mercury poisoning in 1954. His limbs jerked involuntarily, and as the condition progressed he experienced convulsions. Saliva ran from his mouth. His speech was unintelligible. No one could identify the disease; not knowing what else to do, his family placed him in an asylum. He lay there, bedridden, until his death two years later.

From 1955 on, Kawamoto himself began to experience numbness in his

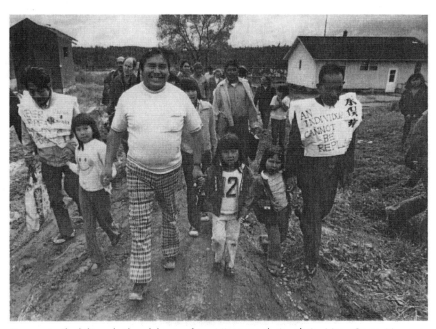

Kawamoto (far left) and other delegates from Minamata during their visit to Grassy Narrows, an indigenous community in Ontario, Canada, also afflicted with mercury poisoning (1975, photo by Shiota Takeshi)

hands and feet, a stiffening of his tongue, and frequent headaches. Combined with fatigue and forgetfulness, these are symptoms of chronic mercury poisoning. Doctors at Minamata Municipal Hospital, not trained in industrial diseases, dismissed Kawamoto's illness as "a cold" or "overwork."[14] Kawamoto's father, who had been a Chisso employee, retired in 1946 and took up fishing; in 1960 he too began showing symptoms of the disease. He was placed in a psychiatric hospital, where he died in 1965. Believing that there must be other patients whose symptoms had gone unrecognized, Kawamoto began to make the rounds of coastal hamlets by bicycle, visiting house after house. In 1966 he earned a nursing license. As a witness to many autopsies, he learned that the brains of those stricken with organic mercury poisoning are atrophied and spongy. Kawamoto never forgave himself for allowing his father to die alone, in a room like a prison cell.[15]

Minamata disease first appeared in fishing villages close to Hyakken Harbor, where Chisso's drainage canal emptied into Minamata Bay. Kawamoto lived in the hamlet of Detsuki, just a five-minute walk from Tsubodan, the neighborhood closest to the effluent gate. Here, one evening in April 1956, five-year-old Tanaka Shizuko's fingers began trembling as she tried to eat. Food fell from her chopsticks. She dropped her bowl. The next morning she could not walk or speak. On the fourth day she lost her sight. Finding no relief for her daughter's agony at local clinics, Shizuko's mother took her to the general hospital, which belonged to the Minamata plant of Chisso Corporation. Ten days later, Shizuko's three-year-old sister Jitsuko developed similar symptoms. Before the children became ill, the mother reported, the family cats had gone mad, emitting terrible cries as they bumped into walls and pillars. On May 1, 1956, Dr. Hosokawa Hajime of the Chisso Factory Hospital submitted a report to the Public Health Office in Minamata describing an unknown disease marked by symptoms characteristic of brain damage, polio, and cerebral palsy. This day marks the "official discovery" of Minamata disease.

Already suffering the critical illness of their children, the Tanakas also had to face the fear and hostility of their neighbors. They were forced to walk back roads and trails. The city sprayed their house with disinfectant, hoping to keep the disease from spreading. "We were ostracized by the villagers," recalls the oldest sister, Ayako. "When we went shopping, we couldn't hand over our money. The shopkeepers would take it with chopsticks or a bowl. People pinched their noses and held their breath as they ran by our house. No one would speak to us." When other villagers showed symptoms of mercury poisoning, they tried to attribute their sickness to different causes. Only the Tanaka family have "*kibyo*, the strange disease," they would say.

Because this was the first time a population had been poisoned through the food chain, local doctors and scientists did not know what they were seeing. The public believed Minamata disease to be a contagious illness of the lowest stratum of society. After three years of agony, Shizuko died in Kumamoto University Hospital. Her parents and grandparents also died of mercury poisoning. Jitsuko, barely able to move or communicate, still lives in the care of her older sister, Tanaka Ayako, who also has symptoms of the disease. "We have reached the bottom," says Ayako. "We cannot be brought down any further."[16]

Dr. Harada Masuzumi, who has dedicated his entire career to helping Minamata disease patients, first visited Minamata in 1961, after graduating from Kumamoto Medical School. "What struck me most deeply," recalled Dr. Harada over three decades later, "was not the physical pain the victims suffered, nor their extreme poverty, but the pain they bore in their hearts due to the treatment they received from neighbors, relatives, employers, and society at large."[17]

Until August 1958, Chisso pumped wastes into Hyakken Harbor, south of the Minamata plant. After damage to the local fishery became more severe and illness among people more widespread, Chisso secretly began, in September, to pump waste into the mouth of the Minamata River to the north. Carried out by the currents, the mercury spread even farther.[18] One year later in Meshima, north of the Chisso plant, Masato's father, Ogata Fukumatsu, a local boss of the Shiranui net fishing industry, began to lose his ability to walk. As methyl mercury attacked his central nervous system Fukumatsu experienced numbness in his hands and feet, loss of coordination, excessive salivation, and disturbances in speech, sight, and hearing, all of which built up to frequent and severe convulsions. The only release from this agony was death. Masato's father died of acute mercury poisoning in late November 1959.

If Minamata disease was "officially discovered" on May 1, 1956, why did it continue to spread, unchecked? In August 1956, Kumamoto University School of Medicine dispatched its first team of investigators. A detailed record was kept of each patient's condition, but it was not until July 1959, after extensive research and experimentation, that the medical team determined conclusively that the illness was caused by organic mercury entering the sea from Chisso's Minamata plant.

That same month Chisso's physician, Dr. Hosokawa, who had dealt with some of the earliest cases of the disease, began to conduct his own experiments. When cat number 400 exhibited the same symptoms he found in his human patients, he sent samples of its brain tissue to Kyushu University for analysis. The tissue showed loss of cerebellum cells characteristic of Minamata disease. Hosokawa reported the results to Chisso executives, who ordered him to stop his experiments and keep silent.[19] On October 7, 1959, the same day Hosokawa's cat developed Minamata disease, Chisso claimed that "Minamata disease may be caused by explosives dumped into the bay by the defunct Japanese Army."[20]

By summer 1959 the desperate pleas of local fishers began to attract media attention. Mediation committees stacked in favor of Chisso gave the local and regional fishing cooperatives no alternative but to accept paltry compensation packages.[21] Chisso promised to install wastewater treatment equipment, but as workers later testified, the pipes conveying waste from the acetaldehyde process were never connected to the treatment system.[22] On December 30 Chisso made one more show of compassion by presenting patients with its infamous "Sympathy (*mimaikin*) Agreement." The agreement stipulated that three hundred thousand yen ($833 at 360 yen/dollar) would be given to a family with a deceased victim, and that annual pensions of one hundred thousand yen ($277) for adults and ten thousand yen ($27) for children would be provided for living victims. Article 5B—annulled by a court ruling in 1973—stipulated that the patients were to relinquish their claims to further compensation even should it be determined that Minamata disease was caused by Chisso's wastes.[23] As far as Chisso management was concerned, the Condolence Agreement of December 30, 1959, marked the closure of the Minamata incident.

Even as Chisso tried to erase Minamata disease from the public mind, Ishimure Michiko (born 1927), an aspiring poet from Minamata, began to record the images that fill the pages of her first book, *Kugai jodo, waga Minamata-byo* (Paradise in the Sea of Sorrow: Our Minamata Disease).[24] Published first in a local journal and then in book format in 1969, Ishimure's poetic documentary became one of the strongest forces in educating the public about the personal and social impact of Minamata disease. Her words attracted a network of professionals and other citizens to aid patients and their families.

Ishimure's profiles of individuals, families, and communities gave Minamata disease a personal face. In her 1964 visit to the Ezuno family, for example, Ishimure provides a glimpse of one of the early sufferers of congenital Minamata disease, Mokutaro, born in 1955. Moku's father is afflicted by mercury poisoning in his thirties, after which Moku's mother abandons the family, leaving the care of the household to her elderly in-laws. Moku's grandfather tells Ishimure, "Parents and siblings generally change a person's diapers only in infancy and at death. Eventually both of Moku's brothers will have to marry; then he'll be a nuisance. . . . I don't have long to live. It's not that I would like to hold death off for my own sake, but I would like to keep living for Moku."[25] Today "Moku," whose real name is Hannaga Kazumitsu, lives in Meisuien, a "rehabilitation center" for Minamata disease patients. Although he has almost no control of his limbs and cannot hold his head upright, he can maneuver through the halls of his daily world in an electric wheelchair.[26]

Organic mercury is conveyed to a fetus both through the umbilical cord and through the placenta. Pregnant women who had reported feeling much better while they carried their child were horrified to learn that the fetus had absorbed the mercury in their bodies. As with adults, the condition of congenital Minamata disease patients differed from person to person. Some children had symptoms similar to cerebral palsy; some were born with varying degrees of mental retardation. Many were unable to walk, feed themselves, or speak; some were unable to hear or see. Many died at a young age. For those still living, the idea that Minamata disease was "over" by 1960 or has been brought to a conclusion today is a mockery of all they have endured.

Masato's nephew, Kosaki Tatsuzumi, was born in 1959, the same year that Ogata Fukumatsu, his maternal grandfather, died of acute mercury poisoning. At the time no one made the connection between Tatsuzumi's condition and Fukumatsu's illness. It never occurred to the family that they would be affected by a disease that had broken out down the coast in Minamata. Later they realized that though their hamlet might be isolated from the road and rail system, both fish and fishermen traveled freely through the Shiranui Sea. The family first took Tatsuzumi to a doctor when they realized he could not hold his head upright. The diagnosis was infantile paralysis. When Tatsuzumi reached school age he was re-examined and certified as a Minamata disease patient.[27]

In 1965 a second mercury poisoning incident occurred in Niigata, along the western coast of northern Honshu. A chemical plant owned by Showa Denko had dumped untreated effluent containing mercury into the Agano River. Six hundred people were affected, over seventy of whom died. The resulting outcry forced the government to admit, in September 1968, that Chisso bore responsibility for Minamata disease. By this time, however, all of the chemical plants in Japan manufacturing acetaldehyde and using mercury as a catalyst had ceased to operate.[28]

In order to cooperate with the Niigata victims, Minamata sufferers, under the leadership of Ishimure Michiko, established the Citizens' Council for Minamata Disease Countermeasures. For the first time Minamata disease victims saw their fellow residents offering a helping hand.[29] Because traditional Japanese society values community prosperity above individual rights, and because Chisso dominated the regional economy, it took great courage for victims to speak for themselves and for other residents to play active roles on their behalf.

The Minamata movement eventually became factionalized, with some groups appealing directly to Chisso and some groups pursuing litigation. In the process, victims received increased outside support but were also broken down physically and emotionally during three decades of appeals and counterappeals. Outside support came primarily from leftist university students disillusioned with Japan's blind pursuit of rapid economic growth, but also from professionals such as doctors, lawyers, engineers, journalists, and photographers. The late American photographer W. Eugene Smith brought wrenching images of Minamata victims to the Western world, but at the price of his health and eyesight. In January 1972, when he was photographing a demonstration at Chisso's plant in Goi, Chiba Prefecture, he was severely beaten by Chisso-hired thugs.

On June 14, 1969, one patient group, representing forty-one victims, entered the litigation process for the first time, filing a damage suit against Chisso in the Kumamoto District Court.[30] Factory workers began to document work-site injuries and deaths from explosions, acid burns, and exposure to excessive heat and toxicants. Dr. Hosokawa, who had resigned from Chisso in 1962, provided testimony from his hospital bed for the first Minamata trial in 1970. When Chisso had negotiated with fishermen and patients in 1959, he disclosed, management had been fully aware that their effluent was the cause of Minamata disease.[31] On March 20, 1973, the court held Chisso guilty of professional negligence. In the judge's words, "The defendant's guiding philosophy of placing profit first and human welfare last is the fundamental cause of Minamata disease."[32] Chisso was ordered to pay the plaintiffs consolation money (isharyo) of sixteen to eighteen million yen each. With this payment, Chisso considered itself "finished" with this group of patients.

Many victims had declined to join in the lawsuit, and instead sought compensation through a government-appointed certification board. Chisso and the prefectural government had established an elaborate certification system. In order to receive compensation from Chisso, Minamata disease sufferers were required to demonstrate five years' residence on the Shiranui Sea coast and submit results of a medical examination to a government-appointed board of doctors. The prefectural governor issued the final determination in each instance.[33]

The complex nature of the certification system and criticism from family or community members discouraged potential applicants, and the majority of patients who did apply were turned down by the board or the governor. The prefecture was pumping money into Chisso at low rates of interest, and the government-appointed board was being encouraged to certify as few applicants as possible. Indications of a possible third outbreak of mercury poisoning in May 1973 along the Ariake Sea coast north of Minamata drew increased public attention and support, and it promoted a rush of new applicants. Bureaucratic wheels turned ever more slowly, and the system became clogged.

It is at this juncture that Kawamoto Teruo organized the Minamata Disease Certification Applicants' Council to develop ways to streamline the process and to encourage patients to apply for certification. Masato joined the newly formed council in 1974 and, inspired by Kawamoto, became deeply involved in the Minamata movement. The movement made its base camp at Minamata Disease Center Soshisha, a support facility established in 1974 with funds donated from all over Japan, including ten thousand dollars from the Ramon Magsaysay Prize (from the Philippines) awarded to Ishimure Michiko for her literary achievements.

Rowing the Eternal Sea follows Masato's activities in the movement, and his sudden resignation from the council in 1985, when the endless pursuit of responsibility and compensation begin to lose meaning, ultimately driving him to "madness" and a spiritual quest for another kind of world. Rejecting the high-speed, plastic society that has filled his sea with nonbiodegradable trash, Masato builds a wooden rowboat, which he names *Tokoyo,* "Eternal World." Although it seems that his destination may be *higan,* the "Other Shore," Masato finds that it is still possible to find paradise within this life. As Ishimure points out at the end of her prologue, we tend to follow, almost unconsciously, whatever direction in which society or our political economy may lead us. It is only when disaster shakes our foundations that we are forced out of our complacency and motivated to reassess the course we have taken.

Following World War II, the Japanese viewed smoke rising from industrial stacks as a symbol of their country's economic rebirth. By the mid-1960s, however, attitudes began to undergo a radical change, brought about in large part by media coverage of victims' movements (*higaisha undo*) and pollution trials issuing from three major incidents: Minamata disease; Yokkaichi asthma, pulmonary diseases resulting from high sulfur oxide emissions; and "*Itai itai*" (it hurts, it hurts) disease, resulting from chronic cadmium poisoning. The year 1970, though bringing little relief to the Minamata patients, was dubbed *kogai gannen,* "the first year of the pollution era." The sixty-fourth session of the Diet in 1970, the so-called environment session, enacted fourteen laws related to pollution control. The Environment Agency (Kankyo-cho) was established in 1971; in 2001 it became a ministry.

How deep was this apparent shift in attitude, and what role did the government play in cleaning up Minamata Bay? It is estimated that over a period of thirty-six years, Chisso released four hundred to six hundred tons of mercury into the bay.[34] Some of the sludge containing more than 25 ppm of mercury was dredged. Fifty-eight hectares (143 acres) of the bay have been filled, in order to bury mercury-laden sediments. In 1974 Kumamoto Prefecture placed dividing nets at the mouth of Minamata Bay (leaving a gap for boat traffic), in an attempt to contain contaminated fish. Members of the fishing cooperative were paid to catch the fish, which they disposed of in metal containers. A sign was posted warning against sport fishing, but a ban was never enforced, for to make it a matter of law would be to assume legal responsibility for the pollution. In July 1997 the bay was declared safe and the nets removed. No species of fish now exceeds the national standard of 0.3 ppm methyl mercury.[35]

In 1996, four decades after the official discovery of Minamata disease, a Compromise Settlement (*Wakai Kyotei*)—popularly known as "the Final Settlement"—was reached between the national government and uncertified Minamata disease sufferers, whereby ten thousand would be eligible for a onetime, lump-sum compensation of 2.6 million yen each. In addition, the sum of 4.94 billion yen was to be divided among five victims' groups to cover legal fees and other expenses incurred over the years.[36] The agreement does not acknowledge those receiving compensation as "Minamata disease patients" but refers to them simply as "those persons who have unavoidable circumstances, *yamuoenu jijo ga aru hito*."[37] The victims agree not to press further charges against, or request further compensation from, Chisso. To follow, at least in form, Japan's "polluter pays principle" (PPP), all payments are channeled through Chisso. With this settlement politically mediated at the national level, the nation declared Minamata disease to be over, once and for all, without ever clarifying the source of moral and legal responsibility.

Since 1978 the national and prefectural governments have provided Chisso with financial support, by issuing prefectural bonds. In the public's view, Chisso has evolved from a private company into a quasi-governmental enterprise.[38] Under the terms of the Final Settlement, the public pays the polluter so that the polluter may in turn pay its victims, the public. Chisso's total budget for treatment of methylated mercury effluents from its Minamata acetaldehyde plant was 1.5 million yen ($4,167); this renovation of the treatment system took place in 1968, shortly before the company stopped producing acetaldehyde.[39] Responsible business practices would have saved lives, communities, the environment, and an enormous drain of public funds. Nevertheless, the Japanese government continues to take the position that in pursuing policies that create a rich country (measured in terms of gross domestic product and urban materialism), it is only natural that some people will be sacrificed. As the government sees it, all that need be done to restore social equilibrium is dole out compensation.[40] If what the patients seek is compassion, a sense that society and the state share in their pain, they have not received it at the national or prefectural levels.

What changes have taken place at the local level, in Minamata itself? At a memorial service for Minamata disease sufferers held on May 1, 1994, Minamata mayor Yoshii Masazumi became the first government representative to offer an apology for the Minamata disease incident. He summed up his address with the words, "I proclaim this day the beginning of a reunification of Minamata's citizens—let us moor together again, as boats in a harbor, that our hearts may be reconciled." Some of the Final Settlement funds were directed toward the establishment of "reconciliation centers," to bring together the various factions of Minamata disease patients, as well as non-patient residents, for discussions and activities that would heal the wounds of decades and set a new direction for the city.[41] Minamata disease—once a taboo subject—is being actively discussed in the schools; it was recently the subject of a high school play. Student groups meet with Minamata disease survivors to hear their life stories.[42]

The population of Minamata has fallen from 46,233 at its height in the sixties to approximately thirty-two thousand today. Six hundred seventy people work directly for Chisso, less than half the former employee number, and another 1,500 work in Chisso-related enterprises.[43] Everyone has endured so much that there is tremendous energy to work together to create a better future. The town administration believes that the regeneration of Minamata must begin with the environment. Minamata now emphasizes "green" tourism; the land reclaimed from the most polluted section of the bay has been declared an "eco-park."

One idea behind green tourism is that the region itself is an eco-museum, a place where we can learn about the relationship between human culture and a specific environment. A movement has grown around the principle of *jimotogaku*, "learning about one's native place." This learning involves becoming more aware of local fauna and flora, listening to local elders, and learning by hands-on experience about traditional farming, gathering, and fishing, as well as rediscovering local cultural history. It is only through an intimate knowledge of place that residents can formulate ecologically sound policy.[44] Environmental efforts include an elaborate trash-separation and recycling process.

Certainly these endeavors have great potential merit, but Masato challenges residents to go beyond recycling and green tourism to consider the broader effects of their continuing lifestyles.

> Today the word "environmentalism" reverberates throughout the world, becoming a buzz word of modern society. Environmental movements promote the separation of garbage, recyling, ecotourism, and renewable energy. I approve of each one of these efforts, and yet they invite my skepticism. I feel that they divert our eyes from the core issues, allowing us to be satisfied with superficial solutions. They enable us to deceive ourselves. Participants develop the attitude that issues of life and nature are to be dealt with solely as technological problems and as part of movements within the system. As we focus on minute measurements such as picograms and parts per million, we tend to forget the larger picture. We all must acknowledge our dependence on modern civilization and technology. We talk about a global crisis, but at the crux of this crisis is our own lack of awareness of how we are affecting other living creatures, how we, as individuals, live our daily lives. Minamata disease constantly shows a new face, whether it be the human population explosion, over-use of pesticides, or nuclear proliferation.[45]

The Minamata incident is but one episode in the ongoing saga of industrial pollution and the larger modernization enterprise. Minamata disease lies latent in the human condition, reaching epidemic proportions wherever the battle cries of "development" and "economic growth" are used to disguise personal greed and indifference to the suffering of others.

A striking Western parallel to the experience of Minamata sufferers may be found in the treatment of miners working in the St. Lawrence Corporation fluorspar mines during the 1940s and 1950s. Poverty-stricken men in the tiny villages along Newfoundland's south coast left a declining fishery to eke out a living in the mines, only to succumb, one after another, to pulmonary diseases and cancers resulting from daily exposure to radiation and silica dust in a largely unregulated industry.

Just as outsiders accused Minamata disease victims of pretending to be sick in order to obtain compensation, upper-level employees of the St. Lawrence Corporation and their families accused the miners of "faking it." "They make up their diseases," said an executive's son.[46] Also, as was the case in Minamata, not only did no one from the St. Lawrence Corporation ever visit miners laid off with fatal diseases, but the firm tried to deny or minimize compensation payments. "A Company is not a poor person, are they?" questioned one widow. "They get lots. And they're making plenty of money from that mine now. I wish the mine had never opened."[47]

Like Ogata Masato, victims of industrial diseases worldwide question the meaning of "compensation" and search for the source of social responsibility. From Minamata to Newfoundland, the sacrifice of people and places calls for a reassessment of the social and environmental costs of irresponsible industrial production, of the implications and limitations of compensation, and of our notions of obligation and responsibility. These are issues that must be considered on an international, national, corporate, and personal level. Masato's personal quest leads to his discovery of "the Chisso within."

Masato's story begins with the vibrant village of his birth and culminates with the possibility of return, if not to the exact place of one's birth, then to a spiritual community, to a consciousness that we owe our existence to the web of interrelationships that constitute life. When we turn full circle, explains Masato, we find ourselves again at the water's edge, a place where all life gathers.[48] This is the launching point for *Tokoyo,* boat of the "Eternal World"—a world defined at once by the past, present, and future; a state of mind, in which we are both Self and Other, responsible not only for our own actions but for those of our society and our species.

NOTES

The translator would like to thank Richard Nelson, Mark and Kyoko Selden, and Michael Taylor for editorial comments, and Ori Arisa of Soshisha for assisting with research and for her warm hospitality.

1. All names are written in the Japanese style, surname first. However, in the case of Ogata Masato, we will use the given name "Masato," to express the close relationship between informant and writer, and between storyteller and reader.

2. Ogata Masato, personal communication, Minamata, October 15, 1999.

3. Castle town, *jokamachi:* towns that grew up around the headquarters of feudal overlords in the Tokugawa period, 1600–1868.

4. Harada Masazumi, *Minamata ga utsusu sekai* (The World Reflected by Minamata) (Tokyo: Nihon Hyoronsha, 1989), 9.

5. Harada, *Minamata ga utsusu sekai,* 85.

6. Harada, *Minamata ga utsusu sekai,* 14.

7. Kurihara Akira, *Shogen Minamata byo* (Testimony: Minamata Disease) (Tokyo: Iwanami Shoten, 2000), Appendix: Minamata byo kanren Nenpyo (Chronology of Minamata disease), 1.

8. Ui Jun, "Minamata Disease," in *Industrial Pollution in Japan* (Tokyo: United Nations University Press, 1992), 108.

9. Iijima Nobuko, ed., *Pollution Japan: Historical Chronology* (Tokyo: Asahi Evening News, 1979), 85, 87; Ui, "Minamata Disease,"106.

10. Timothy S. George, *Minamata: Pollution and the Struggle for Democracy in Postwar Japan* (Cambridge, Mass.: Harvard University Asia Center, 2001), 303. The most comprehensive study of the Minamata incident available in English, this book is highly recommended for readers seeking a deeper understanding of the complexities of this issue.

11. Kurihara, *Shogen Minamata byo,* 12.

12. Harada, *Minamata ga utsusu sekai,* 24.

13. "State held liable for Minamata disease." The Japan Times Online (April 28, 2001), http://www.japantimes.co.jp/cgi-bin/getarticle.p15 (May 5, 2001). A total of 2,995 patients have been certified; 16,143 applicants have been rejected.

14. Kurihara, *Shogen Minamata byo*, 92.

15. Kurihara, *Shogen Minamata byo*, 99.

16. Kurihara, *Shogen Minamata byo*, 29–41.

17. Harada, *Minamata ga utsusu sekai*, 22.

18. A survey conducted by the Kumamoto Health Research Center in 1960 found that while the average Japanese had two parts per million (ppm) mercury in their hair, the hair of residents in the circumference of the Shiranui Inland Sea registered up to 920 ppm. Kurihara Akira, *Shogen Minamata byo*, 99.

19. Mishima Akio, *Bitter Sea: The Human Cost of Minamata Disease* (Tokyo: Kosei, 1992), 48.

20. Iijima, *Pollution Japan*, 148.

21. George, *Minamata*, 79–101.

22. Mishima, *Bitter Sea*, 49.

23. Soshisha Minamata Disease Center, ed., *E de miru Minamata byo* (Illustrated Minamata Disease), in English and Japanese (Yokohama: Seori Shobo, 1993), 58; Ui, "Minamata Disease," 113.

24. Ishimure's book has been translated in full by Livia Monnet, under the title *Paradise in the Sea of Sorrow* (Kyoto: Yamaguchi, 1990).

25. Ishimure Michiko, *Kugai jodo waga Minamata byo* (Pure Land Poisoned Sea, Our Minamata Disease) (Tokyo: Kodansha, 1972), 160–82. Translated in Karen Colligan-Taylor, *The Emergence of Environmental Literature in Japan* (New York: Garland, 1990), 295–309.

26. Personal visits with Hannaga Kazumitsu, Minamata, May 1989 and May 1993.

27. Kurihara, *Shogen Minamata byo*, 168–71.

28. Harada Masazumi, "Minamata Disease as a Social and Medical Problem," *Japan Quarterly* 25, no. 1 (1978): 27.

29. Mishima, *Bitter Sea*, 68–69.

30. George, *Minamata*, 197.

31. Mishima, *Bitter Sea*, 48–49; Iijima, *Pollution Japan*, 292.

32. Soshisha, *E de miru Minamata byo*, 145.

33. Soshisha, *E de miru Minamata byo*, 67.

34. Soshisha, *E de miru Minamata byo*, 30.

35. Minamata Disease Municipal Museum and Minamata Disease Museum, *Ten Things to Know about Minamata Disease* (Minamata Environmental Creation Development Project, 1997), 6.

36. Kurihara, *Shogen Minamata byo*, "Nenpyo," 8; Tokio Marine, "Minamata Victims Accept Government Plan," *Environmental Newsletter* 57 (November 1995), http://www.tokiomarine.co.jp/e0300/html/EnvNov95-2.html#A (October 2, 1999). The term *wakai* refers to a court-mediated, out-of-court settlement.

37. Kurihara, *Shogen Minamata byo*, 109.

38. Zaidanhojin Minamatabyo Sentaa Soshisha, *Gonzui* 50 (February 1999): 16. *Gonzui* is a monthly publication of the Minamata Disease Center Soshisha.

39. Ui, "Minamata Disease," 182, and personal communication, June 18, 2001.

40. Kurihara, *Shogen Minamata byo*, 17.

41. *Gonzui* 49 (November 1998): 3–7.

42. Ori Arisa, personal communication, Minamata Disease Center Soshisha, October 15, 1999.

43. Ori Arisa, personal communication, October 15, 1999. It should be noted that although its Minamata plant has been downsized, Chisso now has plants in Okayama, Shiga, Fukuoka, and Chiba Prefectures, as well as overseas ventures in New York, Hong Kong, and in Guangzhou and Shanghai in China. In August 1998 the Manhattan facility of Chisso America, Inc., was cited by the U.S. Environmental Protection Agency (EPA) for violations of the Toxic Substance Control Act (TSCA). EPA Region 2, "EPA Cites Chisso America, Inc. for Toxic Substance Violations," http://www.epa.gov/region02/epd/98103.htm (October 28, 2000).

44. *Gonzui* 58 (May 2000): 3–7.

45. Oiwa Keibo, transcription of interviews with Ogata Masato, fall 1999. See also *Gonzui* 50 (February 1999): 15–19. Masato criticizes Soshisha for aligning with the local government in efforts to make Minamata a model environmental city. In so doing, he says, Soshisha has distanced itself from Minamata disease sufferers. There are many opinions regarding the role Soshisha should play in the "post-settlement" era.

46. Elliott Leyton, *Dying Hard: The Ravages of Industrial Carnage* (Toronto: McClelland and Stewart, 1975), 134. Another industrial calamity, closer to home, may be found in the history of Love Canal, New York. Lois Marie Gibbs, a resident of the housing complex built on this chemical disposal site, has written extensively about the incident, including *Love Canal: The Story Continues* (Stony Creek, Conn.: New Society, 1998).

47. Leyton, *Dying Hard*, 132–33.

48. Kurihara, *Shogen Minamata byo*, 25.

Prologue

"Out to the Mythological Sea"

Ishimure Michiko

Masato grew bashful as he confided to me, "I've had a wooden boat made, you know. But I haven't told anyone in the village yet." I sensed that something very complex had been taking place in his heart since he had withdrawn his application to be certified as a Minamata disease patient.

A young member of the local patient support group had come up to me and said, "I heard that Masato fell while setting nets to catch red snapper. When I went to see him, his legs and arms were stretched out in convulsions. It's pretty unnerving to actually watch someone in this state."

Now, as I gazed at Masato, his eyes blinking peacefully, I felt that he must be close to getting back on his feet again. He inspired me with awe.

As I sat there chatting with him, I learned something quite shocking. He said that he could not remember once seeing a wooden sailboat. All boats today seem to be made of plastic, he said. I had no idea. Were all those boats floating in the bay made of plastic? I realized that some must be plastic, but I had imagined that the majority were made of wood. I was shaken by my own ignorance. So Japan had come to this?

My mind wandered to the piles of old craftsmen's tools that I frequently saw in secondhand shops. Rusting away among household electronic appliances were the large saws and axes of lumberjacks, the planes and squares of carpenters, the various trowels used by plasterers, the iron tongs of blacksmiths, and the chisel and hammer of stone masons. Among these there must also have been the adz of a boat builder.

"You were lucky to find a traditional boat builder," I said.

"Yes. I asked the owner of a boat factory, whose father had been friends with my father, if he knew of someone. He introduced me to a boat maker who still remembered the old ways. When I approached him about a wooden boat, he was astonished. After all, you won't find anyone nowadays making

17

a boat out of wood. As we talked, though, he took me seriously and accepted the order. It was Chisso that first produced plastic goods in our region. None of these things, not even the boats, seem any different to me than the garbage I find drifting at sea."

Even though we might look at them as one more kind of nonbiodegradable trash, I suppose we must acknowledge that these plastic boats are indispensable for commercial fishing today. Still, I deeply sympathized with Masato's desire to have a boat of wood, even if it is far less resilient than a boat of fiberglass and plastic.

There are some places that only a wooden boat can take you.

"Would you be willing to paint on the name for me? It's '*Tokoyo*.' "

Ah, *tokoyo*—the "Eternal World"—so that's where you're headed, I thought. This was a man whose entire extended family had been in the grip of death. I put my soul into the calligraphy, but I felt the characters lacked confidence.

I was surprised, some time later, to receive a letter of invitation to the boat's launching. We followed the shoreline north toward Masato's village and stopped at the small fishing hamlet of Odomari, in the village of Tsunagi. From the shipyard you could look over toward the hot-spring resort of Yunoko. It was May.

Wrapped in the scent of fresh wood, Masato's small boat seemed ideal for a voyage to the Eternal World.

"Please come aboard," invited Masato's elder brother-in-law.

I hesitated, mindful of the traditional taboo that excludes women from boat-launching ceremonies, but Sugimoto Yu and his wife Eiko encouraged me to board.[1]

"Why not? Let's get on. Hurry now, hurry."

We had to launch the boat on the rising tide, and if we wasted any more time the tide would go out. As the bow hit the water, golden threads of light spread in all directions, rippling out to sea. On a hill jutting into the ocean, a cluster of chinquapin trees emanated a solemn glow.

Where is this "Eternal World," anyway? I wondered. Perhaps it's a place where the image of rebirth into a better world is ever present . . . a place where even death is softly illuminated by the life in trees and grass. I needn't worry. Masato will surely return.

The bow of our small boat tumbled defiantly over the waves, heading toward the sea as it was before the outbreak of Minamata disease, and even farther into the ocean of the distant past. As I looked over the bow, which was shaped like the topknot of a woman's traditional hairstyle, I tried to imagine the many years of hardship that Masato and the Sugimotos had

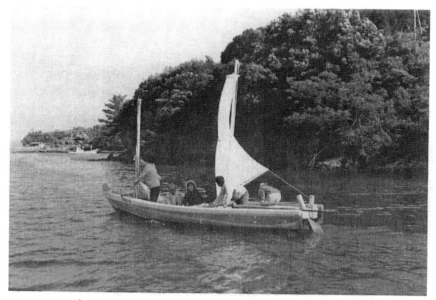

A boat ride for guests after the launching of Tokoyo *in May 1987.*
Writer Ishimure Michiko sits in the center, wearing a hat.

endured as victims of Minamata disease. Needless to say, I could not grasp even a single day of their suffering.

Masato lifted a large platter, scattering rice and salt in the waves as an offering to the sea. The Sugimotos pointed to a plate full of sliced raw fish. The men began dipping the *sashimi* in salt and eating it. Then, they scooped up sardines swimming about in the fish box and put them in their mouths, looking toward the horizon. The sardines darted about in the mouths that held them.

"They're fresh, all right!"

Each step of the ceremony came as a surprise. The boat launching was a ritual in which the lives of the ocean, people, and fish all merged vibrantly. As we headed toward the open sea, I looked up at Masato, my heart singing praises to the gods. He was excitedly holding the rope that controlled the sail, trying to follow the instructions of the more experienced men.

Everyone on board was staring far ahead, as if lost in the thoughts welling up inside. The boat plunged onward, bearing its cargo of rich silence. I was told that the wind was blowing from the east.

After we rounded three points and approached the anchorage at Masato's village, I saw boats in the harbor gathering to meet us. There must have been twenty of them, and judging from the straight line of their advance and their speed, I realized that they were not wooden sailboats but modern powered craft made of plastic. Our boat must have stood out, even from afar. I had a sense of heightened anticipation.

Gradually we drew closer to shore. This cluster of houses, which I had previously approached only by land, peacefully clung to the shoreline along the curve of the anchorage. Doors opened, and people streamed out, looking and pointing in our direction as they headed for the breakwater. It looked like the entire hamlet must be there. I wished I were close enough to hear their words. What was Masato feeling just now?

Closely escorted by the other boats, we pulled up to the dock. Soon we could distinguish individual faces. I can see them before me even now, those looks of quiet admiration that seemed to say, "Oh, so this is the kind of boat that Masato built." Although Masato had intended to keep the boat a secret, the villagers had probably known about it all along. For his sake, however, they had kindly feigned ignorance.

The rich silence I had experienced earlier on the boat now spread to the crowd awaiting us at the dock. It was in this atmosphere that the *Eternal World* reached the shore. The fiberglass boat that reached us first pulled up alongside. The captain caressed the gunwale of our wooden boat and whispered quietly, as if sharing a secret, "Well done. Yes. It's a beauty."

The captain from the next boat jumped aboard and touched the sail, examining it closely. Careful not to seem too intrusive, he spoke casually. "It's not set quite right." He gave Masato the name of a friend. The problem could be fixed in no time at all, he added. Later I was told that "set" referred to the amount of play in the sail when filled out by the wind.

The villagers were reserved, but they couldn't hide their excitement as they drew closer, wanting to touch this boat that exuded the scent of fresh wood. It was as if they had gathered to praise a newborn baby.

Masato seemed to be totally absorbed, but he stepped onto land saying that he had promised a boat ride to his nephew. This nephew, Tatsuzumi, who had been born with Minamata disease and was severely disabled, was on the breakwater waiting in his wheelchair, surrounded by family members. Tatsuzumi was an attractive young man, despite his disabilities. After some time passed, Masato returned to the boat with an air of disappointment.

"He says he's afraid, because he's never ridden in a boat before. We'd made plans, and he was looking forward to it, but . . ."

A man nearby spoke up. "So Tatsuzumi says he's afraid, does he? Hmm." Everyone sighed sympathetically.

Here was a man who had been raised in a fishing family and was close to thirty; yet he was afraid of the ocean and of boats. Masato and Tatsuzumi were close to the same age, and no doubt the villagers had affectionately watched these two grow up together on their native soil, where all shared the same destiny. I knew that Masato was the youngest of twenty brothers and sisters. I felt that his family was blessed with genuine kindness.

Our wooden boat, like a sacred object in a ritual as yet unknown to us, rocked gently on the water, enveloped by the gaze of these kind men and women. At noon there was an outburst of activity as a feast began. The manager of the shipyard, a large man, began singing a local folk song in such a strong, free-spirited voice that it must have carried all the way to the Amakusa Islands, across the bay.

How I remember that day.

The Shiranui Sea, having experienced unprecedented suffering, is beginning to regenerate, assuming a mythical quality.

And Masato's small wooden boat, entrusting itself to the light of the sun and the moon, has pointed its prow and raised its sail, bravely heading straight into the collective unconscious that comprises the sum total of human "progress and enlightenment."

TRANSLATOR'S NOTE

1. Sugimoto Eiko was born in 1938. She grew up in Modo, where her father was a boss of the local net fishery, employing thirty to forty people. In 1958 Eiko's mother, a cheerful, healthy woman who had cooked meals for the employees for over thirty years, began complaining of body aches. Once a lively conversationalist, she fell silent. When she became so ill that she no longer felt cooking burns on her body, Eiko's father took his wife to the hospital. That night the local radio station announced that "the strange disease" had broken out in Modo. "My most painful memory," says Eiko, "is the way we were treated by others in the hamlet." Her father's employees left. People cut the family's nets and used their boats without permission. Both Eiko and her husband Yu are now certified Minamata disease patients. Today Eiko, Yu, and one of their sons are captains of sardine boats. The Sugimotos check the mercury content of all their fish and sell them directly in the local market and to supporters throughout the country. Letters of appreciation from distant buyers brighten the Sugimotos' lives. Kurihara Akira, *Shogen Minamata byo* (Tokyo: Iwanami Shoten, 2000), 129–46.

Part One

常世の舟

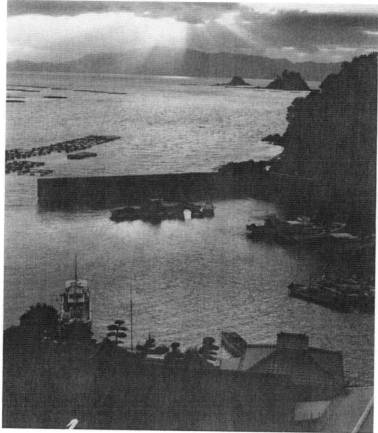

Sunset on the Shiranui Sea viewed from the bluff behind Masato's house. The small building with tiled roof facing the water is ''Yuuan,'' Masato's study. Masato's wooden boat Tokoyo is seen behind the roof. Beyond the sea is a silhouette of the Amakusa Islands.

A Vibrant Village

I was born on November 8, 1953, in the main house of the Ogata clan, about fifty meters from where I live today. In our remote village, tradition still prescribes that the eldest son inherit the main house. As is expected of younger sons, I set up a branch household when I became an adult. Presently the main house is occupied by the eldest son of my eldest brother. It is his responsibility to take care of the assets, cemetery, and ancestral tablets of our clan.

Our village, Oki, is located on a small peninsula called Meshima, meaning "woman island." Directly across the water, the inland sea of Shiranui, is Shimojima, one of the Amakusa Islands. My father's family immigrated to the mainland from Shimojima. It was when grandfather was still young, so it must have been about 120 years ago. Currently there are fifty-seven households in Oki. In all of Meshima there are only two hundred houses, so our village represents about one-fourth of the population. We're one of the oldest families in these parts—not the very oldest, but perhaps next in line. Within the village is a hamlet called Ikenoshiri, consisting of nineteen households. Six of the nineteen houses are referred to as Kochidomari, or "eastern anchorage." This is where I live.

My father, Ogata Fukumatsu, had eighteen children. I was the youngest, born when he was fifty-six. My father married three times. The second marriage lasted only about three months. Apparently the bride fled when she discovered how hard her life would be. With his first wife he had eight girls and four boys. His oldest son died of sickness in the war, so the next oldest became head of the family. After Father's first wife died—an event probably not unrelated to giving birth to so many children—he took my mother as his final wife. Together they had six more kids. I was born when my mother was close to forty. Of her six children, two boys and a girl died shortly after birth. Three are still living. I was the last.

My mother already had two daughters when she married my father. I don't think she had been formally married Those daughters are still living. Count-

25

ing the children who died, there were twenty of us. I was the twentieth, although in the family register I'm listed as the eighteenth.

In my earliest memories, my brothers and sisters were still living at home. We caught all kinds of fish, including red snapper, mullet, and cutlass, but our primary income came from sardines. We used a huge net to catch sardine fry, which would later be sun dried. In those days we didn't have hydraulic rollers to pull in the nets. This was back when most people still used rowboats, and we needed lots of manpower. We'd boil the sardines for a short time, leave them out to dry, and then sell them to a wholesaler.

Our family started out with fixed-shore-net fishing, shifted to trawl netting for sardines, and then moved into purse seining, employing a lot of men. Father was one of seven or eight bosses, *amimoto*, in the village net fishery. Due to mechanization the number gradually decreased, until only one remained. This boss hires mainly family members, so essentially the old "boss" system has vanished.

I had many brothers and sisters, and the brother who succeeded as head of the family had six children. Although most of my sisters were married off by the time I was a small child, the house was full of people who came to work for us. There were also live-in servants who did domestic chores. I remember that two of them were mentally retarded. Among the servants there were also some Koreans. These people eventually left to look for work in the Osaka area, in the late fifties and early sixties. In our heyday we'd have thirty or forty people living and working with us. We also had employees who commuted from neighboring houses and villages.

In sardine fishing a boat would go out ahead to find the fish. Two others followed towing a net. A fourth carried the catch. The boats that needed the greatest number of hands, of course, were those with the nets. Purse seining required about thirty people. They would light a big fire on the edge of the boat at night to attract the fish, and then they would set the net. Right after the war this was the biggest industry in the Shiranui Sea. During the war, most of our hands were drafted, so no one caught many fish. Toward the end of the war, especially, people thought it dangerous to be at sea during a bombing attack. Then the war ended, and everyone came home. The fish stocks were up, and the men were back. This is when purse seining got started, and it remained popular until the late fifties.

Then our region was struck by Minamata disease. Fish stocks dwindled, and we couldn't sell what we did catch. This happened in the early sixties.

When I was small the community was thriving. People would come to work from nearby villages and from the Amakusa Islands. Second and third sons who couldn't inherit farmland from their fathers would come from the countryside to fish. There was even a guy who came all the way from Shikoku to sell kimono fabric and ended up staying here and working for us. The number of households hasn't changed, but there were a lot more people back then. The atmosphere of the village was entirely different. It was vibrant.

As you see, I was born and raised surrounded by lots of people. There was a strong feeling of family, but at home there was no clear-cut distinction between true family and nonfamily members. Many of my sisters ended up marrying employees. It was all very natural—how else would we find suitable mates for so many women?

Imagine the din of more than thirty people eating together! These weren't like meals today, where you can get just about anything you want, but simple affairs consisting of rice mixed with barley, miso soup, and some broiled or boiled fish. When we were really busy, we'd make do with sweet potatoes and rice balls. Even when we'd steam two big pots of rice, there wouldn't be a grain left. Meals were lively and fun, but if you didn't concentrate on eating, you'd be left without anything. The proportion of rice to barley was seven parts to three, or six parts to four. "It was worse than this during the war," my mother would always remind us. She would put rice in a two-liter sake bottle and churn it with a stick to remove the bran. Because we had a big family, she had to do this every day. "That's why my shoulders ache even now," she would complain.

The Bitter Sea

My father was a very strict man. There were lots of hotheaded young men in their teens and twenties in both my family and the village. There was always a fight going on somewhere. These fights usually started after the men had been drinking. Father wouldn't tolerate fights or bullying among his family or workers. Whether it was a family member or an outsider, Father would call them in and berate them in a thundering voice. There were some people who teased the mentally retarded men who worked for us. Calling such a man into the room, Father would poke at the fire in the hearth and, without saying a word, fling the hot fire tongs at the offender. Father was a man of few words, and the offender would be ready to flee the minute he walked in the room.

I saw all of these things very clearly and remember them well, because I was always at his side—either in his lap or right next to him. I probably spent twenty hours a day with him. I was Father's favorite child. At three or four I would quarrel with my sister, who had just entered elementary school. Even if I was to blame, Father would scold my sister. "He's still too small to understand," my father would say, expecting my sister to accept responsibility.

My childhood memories are unusually vivid. I even remember peeing on Father at age two or three, when he was carrying me on his back. By the time I was three my father would take me out in the oar-powered fishing boat. I was also with him when he'd mend the nets. As he boiled sardines, autumn through winter, and even when he went out to cut winter firewood and bring it back by the truckload, I was always at his side. Although he wasn't as talkative as parents are today, my father talked to me quite a bit. He also told me stories and sang folk and popular songs.

Just being near him gave me a sense of security. Thinking about it now, I realize how deeply I admired this man, my father. I'm sure that the respect shown to him by my family and by the villagers also contributed to my own sense of awe. He was stubborn and had no tolerance for what he perceived as wrong. I guess he was typical of the traditional Kumamoto man. Once he

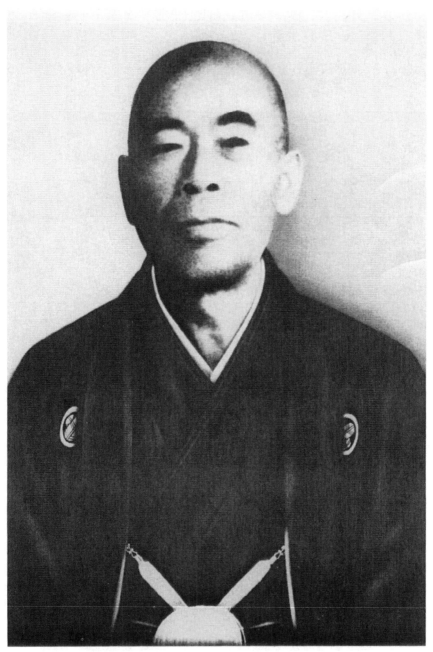

A portrait of Ogata Fukumatsu (1897–1959) taken a few years before his death

had set his mind to something, he would stay right on course and wouldn't be budged. The land on which this house stands today used to be ocean and boulders, but my father reclaimed the area by filling it over ten years with rocks he hauled with his own hands. His body was muscular; he had the legs and arms of a giant.

I can remember my father's daily schedule as if it were yesterday. He would drink *shochu*, a local wine distilled from sweet potatoes, five times a day, one teacup at a time. He preferred to sleep with me, rather than my mother. He awakened very early—about three in the morning. That's when our day would begin. Because we had this routine, I didn't play with other children my own age—at least not while Father was living. I was content just to follow him everywhere. I was with him when he visited farm villages, bringing gifts of fish. I accompanied him to places where they sold nets and to the boat builder's shop. I was at his side when he attended village meetings. I must be the only person of my generation who witnessed those old village meetings.

In those days dolphins were often seen in our coastal waters. I remember the day Father cleaned two of them right here, where I built my study. We salted the meat and stored it in a barrel. I'm sure we must have eaten it for three months straight. It wasn't very tasty, as I recall. As Father was cutting into the meat, I heard him say there were two unborn babies inside. I felt sorry for them and asked him to return them to the sea. Father agreed, and we released them into the water right in front of the house. But since they hadn't been born naturally, they just slowly sank out of sight. For some reason, that scene is still vivid in my mind.

Not even the burliest of the village youths could stand up to my father. He was awesome. He made no distinction between his own children and other kids. There are people in their fifties and sixties in the village today who were once scolded by my father when they were young. Father was very strict with himself, as well. Not a man worked harder. After all, it was his belief that to get more than two hours of sleep a night was a luxury. He was someone who had endured many hardships. Right after he entered elementary school he had lost his mother, and her children did not get along with their new stepmother. They didn't get along with their father—that is, my grandfather—very well, either. Father dropped out of elementary school after two years and went to work at age eight. That's why he could barely read or write.

Once he told me this story. When he was a child he had been approached by some men who invited him to join them on a fishing trip. He would make good money, they promised. He fished with them all the way to the Korean Peninsula, but they never paid him. So, at night, while everyone was sleeping, father would go fishing on his own. In this way he earned enough money for passage home. This must have been around the beginning of the Taisho period (1912–1926). In those days five or six men would row a boat with the help of a small sail. They navigated by the stars. It was because he worked so hard, like this, that he eventually became a boss in the net fishing industry. He told me that the only things he inherited from my grandfather were two baskets, a rice bowl, and a pair of chopsticks. My father would say to me over and over, as if intoning a mantra, "It's a bitter sea out there." He repeated the same phrase to all the young men, speaking of hardships at sea, of work, of life. "Life is hard, so be prepared." This was his message.

I seldom saw my father asleep. Whenever I woke up to pee, he was still awake. He would be sitting by the *irori*, our sunken hearth, absorbed in thought. He was always thinking—not just about tomorrow and the next day but ten years ahead, or perhaps even farther. Every night he sat like that, next to the fire. When we bought new nets, for example, he made his decision based on his plans for the next decade. He never consulted anyone, and he never made mistakes. From the time I was little, he was already making decisions about where I would live thirty or forty years later.

Deep inside my child's heart I cherished the hope that someday I too would become a man like this. He had an incredible presence. At the end of fishing season, when salaries were distributed, or at a village meeting or some other village event, twenty or thirty men might have gathered, making a great commotion. But when it came time to get down to business, my father had only to clear his throat once before the crowd fell silent. He was a man of few words, but what he did say was full of meaning. Even though I was a young child, I somehow understood the weight of his words. His words had dignity, soul. Fuzzy language seems to be the fashion today; words have somehow become empty. Our vocabulary has increased, but these new words are short-lived. Meaningless words flood out of our television sets. My father, on the other hand, didn't waste a single word.

Competing Souls

In autumn we caught *shirogo*, sardine fry. During the winter we caught *ami*, or opposum shrimp, which we salted down before marketing. In spring we would catch grown sardines and other fish. Although the catch might change, fishing continued all year round. In the past you could catch sardine all year; seasonal fish included *konoshiro* (gizzard shad), *bora* (striped mullet), *sayori* (halfbeak), and so on. We prepared different nets according to the fishing spot, season, and type of fish. We fished the entire Shiranui Sea. When we fished with purse seines we even went as far as Akune, in Kagoshima Prefecture. Things like shellfish, sea cucumber, and sea urchins were abundant near the shoreline, where boats were not necessary. Women and children would gather just enough for the family meal. Occasionally sea cucumber and octopus were harvested to sell. Work on both sea and land was shared by everyone, men and women alike. Sometimes women went out fishing. The only time women weren't allowed to board a boat was during a boat-launching ceremony, a custom still observed today. Women would remain on shore, preparing a feast. I never heard a woman complain about it.

On the whole, farming was considered women's work. They grew sweet potatoes, barley, and vegetables. The men were busy mending nets and taking care of the boats. In order to reduce insect and worm damage, the men would collect branches of pine and cedar, burning them with old leaves and needles to creosote the wood. They might also paint the boats. My family grew rice on the acre and a half of paddy land that Father had purchased. Everyone shared the work of transplanting rice seedlings and harvesting the grain. An area that's now a *mikan* orchard used to be the field where we grew crops for our own use. The only things that had to be purchased with cash were foods like salt, sugar, soy sauce, and sake. Orchards of *amanatsu*, or sweet pomelo, became widespread from the mid-1960s. Even though we might buy special dishes for New Year's or *Obon* (All Souls' Day), in mid-August, we would generally barter for goods.

My mother came from the nearby village of Akasaki, which was about evenly divided between those who farmed and those who fished. She grew up in a farming family, and to her, life consisted of no more than growing food and eating it. It would be fair to say that my mother was the exact opposite of my father. Her thoughts were small and her vision narrow. My father used to say to her, "I'll give you a break, so go learn something about society." She didn't think in a rational way. Since I spent my childhood with eyes focused on my father, to me my mother was just someone who worked without saying a word. It wasn't that I clashed with her—that would come later, when I was older.

Traditionally, farmers have felt superior to fishermen and have looked down their nose at them. It was not until after the war, when net fishing for sardines became popular, that the fishing industry blossomed. Until that time fishermen definitely occupied the bottom rung. For one thing, fishermen were very poor, and their lives were unstable. Another reason for the difference in status was that farmers owned real estate, in the form of rice paddies, vegetable fields, and forest land; fishermen did not, with the exception of those like my father, who worked hard to save up their money and bought rice paddies and woodlands. Father was especially keen on forested land. He used to tell us, "Even when it's too stormy to go to sea, our trees are growing taller in the rain." As he accrued forest land and planted trees, he would tell us children, "This is for you." In this way, he was thinking fifty or even a hundred years into the future. I think this is the basic difference between traditional and contemporary people. How many people are there in Japan today who are thinking fifty or a hundred years ahead?

My father caught more fish than anyone else. Almost every year his catch exceeded everybody else's in the fishermen's union. This was, first of all, because he worked harder than anyone else. While others slept, he was up working. Moreover, he had a sixth sense for fishing. As I mentioned before, he would sit at home by the hearth, contemplating many things. But the most important thing on his mind was fishing. I remember him muttering things to the effect that soon there would be a flood tide, which would mean that at such and such a place there were bound to be such and such kinds of fish. They would come close to the shore. Perhaps "thinking" isn't the right term. As he faced the hearth my father seemed to see certain images in front of him. Rather than thinking, he was feeling, or intuiting. This ability still remains to a small extent with my generation. Of course, anyone can catch fish after thinking and planning. But there is definitely another approach, that of "intuiting." I think this power of intuition was especially strong among those born in the Meiji period (1868–1912).

Before the advent of motorized boats, our ancestors would go out to sea for two or three days at a time in rowboats equipped with a cookstove. They would take water, firewood, and rice, and they would bring along straw mats to use as a makeshift roof. They never used the expression "go fishing." They would say simply, "We're heading out to sea." My father often referred to fishing as a game between competing souls. He would explain, for example, "Today the gray mullet were jumping. But we couldn't catch any. Today we lost to the souls of the fish." Sitting beside the hearth, or going out to gaze at the ocean, he was reading the seascape in his mind. He was problem solving. These weren't riddles you could solve by logical thinking. It was a matter of being on the same wavelength with the world of fish. Of course, experience played a critical role, but this wasn't the only factor. Even among fishermen who had been in the business for the same amount of time, the catch would vary significantly. It was a game of competing souls, Father would say.

As times changed, competition between souls disappeared. Modern men use technology to catch fish under almost any conditions. There is no room for intuition, for reading the seascape. The old fishermen didn't just compete with the souls of fish, they also competed with the tides. Today fishermen simply look at a newspaper or at a tide table to determine the time of low and high tide, but in reality tides are not such simple phenomena. High tide, low tide, and slack tide occur at a slightly different time for each given place, and the characteristics of the tides differ as well. Especially in inlets and along the sides of channels, the movements of the tides can be very complex. If you make a mistake, you can find yourself in real trouble. You'll damage your nets.

Incidentally, around here we don't say, "the net is torn." Rather, we say, "the net has been injured," as if it is a living thing. You can see that a lot of water has collected in my boat, *Tokoyo*, tied up in front of the house. In these parts we don't say "water has collected," but rather, "the boat's collecting scum." Whether it be the boat, the net, the tide, or the fish, we treat all of our partners as living things.

In the old days we used to fish even at night. When we were stung by scorpion fish or pinched by crabs, we'd let out a yell, scolding them, "You old scorpion fish," or "Damn you, crab!" Fish, crabs, and men would be engaged in conversation. All things are related, like links in a chain. Though they may not belong to the sphere of humans, we can still communicate with them—fish, cats, dogs. It's painful to realize that we are losing even this sensibility.

Ebisu is the most important god among fisher folk. We offer him *shochu* without fail each day. Some days we pour it over his statue, and sometimes we place it before him in a cup. When you begin building a boat, when you let out a new net for the first time, when you start a new fishing season, you pray to Ebisu. Even when you have a drink of *shochu* on the boat, you first

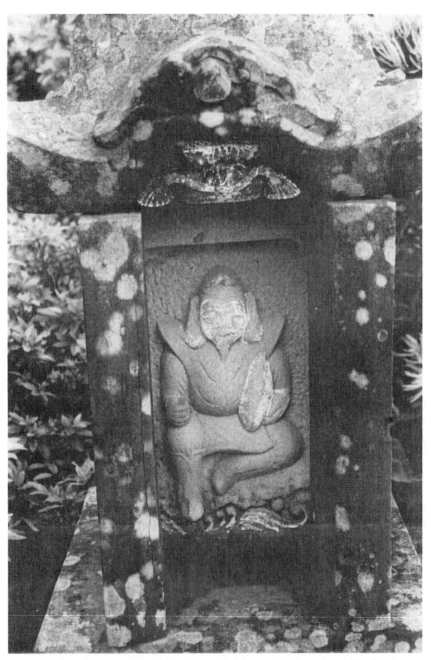

An enshrined stone image of Ebisu-san, god of the sea, in Masato's neighborhood.

toast Ebisu, to show your respect. They say that even a boat has a "boat spirit." There is a special spot in a boat where one of the boards has been hollowed out, and this is where an image representing this spirit is placed. We pray to the boat spirit to protect us from harm, and we pray to the ocean that we may take a lot of fish. We don't have to speak out loud. If we simply utter the name "Ebisu-*san*," with a prayer in our hearts, that's enough. Just intoning his name is strangely calming.

Fishermen try to avoid dropping metal objects, like nuts and bolts, into the water. This is what Ebisu hates most. Another thing he detests is pickled plums. They say that when you drop these things it takes the ocean seven years to push them back up to the shore. We believe that Ebisu is a god who was once banished to sea in the form of a leech-child. A leech has no arms or legs, so it has to pick up everything with its mouth. That's why it takes seven years. It's a lot of work to impose on this god. If you substitute plastic objects and factory effluent for metal objects and pickled plums, you can apply the concept to environmental problems we face today. Imagine how long it would take Ebisu to get rid of them! There probably isn't anyone born five years later than my generation who has even heard of this old wisdom.

When I was a child, there were many village ceremonies and festivals. The biggest events were launching boats and raising house frames. Relatives and acquaintances would all gather to help. Weddings were another big event. In those days, weddings always took place at home. In our hamlet of Ikenoshiri, the eleventh day of January, May, and September by the old lunar calendar were also festive occasions. On these days all nineteen families would get together to share food and drink, each preparing a special dish like *namasu* (pickled meat, fish, and vegetables) and *sashimi*, raw fish. We called it the Eleventh Day Festival. This custom still exists, but instead of holding a pot-luck, each family takes a turn at preparing the meal; instead of the lunar calendar, we use the modern calendar; and instead of having the meal at someone's house, we use the community hall. Everyone in our village used to go by boat to the Suwa Festival in our neighboring town, Sashiki. There was nothing livelier. Children would save all their allowance money for this occasion. And then, of course, there were the festivities held at New Year's and during the week of *Obon* in mid-August, when we welcome home the souls of the deceased. If it weren't for these holidays, we would never have received new clothes.

When I was little, the annual sports day at elementary school also took the form of a festival. Adults and children alike attended. People would get drunk and fight, and the tug-of-war almost became a real war. Everyone blew off steam in this way, during festivals and ceremonies. These events marked the cycle of the year.

Liquor was indispensable at these events. My father, who had many young people working for him, made sure to keep a large supply of sake and *shochu* on his shelves and stored under the floor. He would sit cross-legged on the floor, above the storage space, with a cup of liquor in his hand. Man, could he drink! And yet I never once saw him drunk. Although he would sing folk songs at village feasts, he wasn't the type of person who tried to stir up a crowd. There are always people willing to play this role. Even when drinking my father was always conscious of his obligation to hold the family together. That's why he was strict, and even though he drank, he never let drink get the best of him.

What's Going On?

When there was a big stir around the city of Minamata following the first outbreak of the strange disease, my father dismissed it, saying, "As long as you drink *shochu*, you'll never catch a disease like that." In those days people never even imagined that the sea might be poisoned by chemicals. It was rumored around the port, though, that Chisso looked pretty suspicious. Minamata is often referred to as Chisso's "castle town," a town that has developed around a large company, just as a town might have grown up around a castle in the feudal period. My village is some distance from Chisso, however, so no one here stood to benefit from Chisso's presence. Also, since no one from the neighboring communities commuted to work at Chisso, no one envied this so-called elite group of company employees. Chisso meant nothing to us at all, and we simply ignored the rumors.

Then, my father, the picture of health and vigor, suddenly lost all his energy. He was the first person among all our neighbors and relatives to be afflicted by the disease. I remember that it was around ten o'clock in the morning, on a warm day in September 1959. Father came walking toward us wearing only one straw sandal. I was sitting on a straw mat in the yard, and my mother and sisters were nearby. "I don't know why, but I don't feel well," Father muttered.

"What's wrong?" asked either my mother or my sister.

"My hands are numb," he answered.

They thought he must have caught a cold, but I thought there was something strange in the unsteady way he was standing and walking. Then, as he entered the house, he stumbled on the threshold. From that moment, his condition worsened before our very eyes. We took him right away by boat to the hospital in town. That was the beginning of the end.

Even at the hospital they couldn't figure out what was going on. We were told to return in two or three days. Each day he became worse. By our next visit, he was in such bad shape that he was hospitalized immediately. He was

39

sent from the town clinic to Kumamoto University Hospital for an examination, but even the university doctors couldn't figure out what was going on.

When Father was hospitalized I wanted to stay with him, but his own
desire for me to remain with him was even stronger. At first my mother,
brothers, and sisters would take turns caring for him, but Father missed me
and would ask them to bring me along. So I joined them. I recall that he was
in the hospital for nearly two months, but I was only with him for about half
that time. When I stood up to go to the bathroom, he would ask me where I
was headed. "Just going out to pee," I would reassure him. "I'll be right back."

I was only six, but I sensed that he was going to die. I could see for myself
that in spite of all the injections and medicine he received, he continued to
deteriorate. All the adults, whether it was my mother, my brothers and sisters, or the doctors, seemed at a total loss. Although they wouldn't speak
openly in front of my father, the family would get together in the hall and
consult with each other about moving him to another hospital. I remember
thinking that I too must try to do something for him. When I lit a cigarette
for him, he was really happy. But he didn't want to take all the injections
and medications recommended by the doctor and my brothers and sisters.
Since it was obvious that he wasn't improving, he would complain, "These
quacks are just trying to make money off me!" Just getting this many words
out of his mouth was difficult. My father's words became increasingly unintelligible. Since Mother and I were with him every day, we could figure out
what he was trying to say. But if my brothers and sisters and other visitors
stayed away for as long as week, they could no longer understand him at all.
So I became his interpreter. "What did Dad say?" they would ask me.

My father hated all those shots and pills the doctors gave him. I think it
may have been morphine or some other painkiller. Nothing else had any
effect. Soon my father had become a case study for employees of the Minamata Public Health Department and doctors from Kumamoto University
Hospital. When he tried to stand up and walk, he would fall over. If he managed to take two or three steps, he would bump into a pillar or the wall. He
clawed at the walls and pillars in frustration and pain. He refused to listen to
the doctors, the nurses, or my mother. But he would never oppose anything
that I said to him. No matter how much pain Father was experiencing, he
would try to compose himself in my presence. Because of this, the doctors
and my family would all try to reach him through me. He'll listen to you,
they would say, so please have him take this medicine.

As I look back on those days, I feel that this is what people mean when
they talk about "being tested." As I watched my father's condition worsen
each day, I felt that I had to do something. I would rack my brains for what
that something might be. I did every little thing I could think of—lighting

his cigarettes, giving him his pills, rubbing his back. It wasn't because anyone asked me to. I did it all of my own volition. It wasn't that I was being tested by someone's criticism. I was being tested by the circumstances themselves. "I just have to do something," I thought. In this reaction, a child is no different from an adult.

Nowadays hospitals provide all of the patient's meals, from breakfast to dinner, but back then the patient's family had to prepare them. Mother worked in the kitchen along with the women accompanying other patients. It wasn't like a modern kitchen, simply a room with a dirt floor and a common stove. Each morning the women would light charcoal, to simmer miso soup and roast some mackerel. My mother tried to do all the cooking while my father was asleep. If he awakened while I was out with Mother, he'd feel so lonely that he would cry out for me. Somebody would come down to tell me he was awake, and as soon as I entered the room he would calm down. Sometimes he would tell my mother to go home, but never me.

Father slept only when he was absolutely exhausted. Most of the time the pain kept him awake. At first he would sleep for one or two hours at a time, but soon his sleep became shorter and more erratic; he seemed to go mad. Seeing this, the other patients and their caregivers went out of their way to treat me well. They all knew how hard it was for me. Just to get him to drink soup was a real task. Father shook so violently that only about one-fourth of the bowl would make it down his throat. The rest of it would spill.

Two Hints

It was during that time that I first used cash to buy things. I bought tofu for the miso soup. The store was only two or three buildings from the hospital. At first I went along with my mother. After we'd gone there together a number of times, she sent me out to get some tofu by myself. It was around noon. When I stepped out of the hospital, the road was crowded with people. There was a cross-country race, someone explained. It must have been an event organized by the local youth association, but at the time I had no idea what was happening. I simply followed the crowd and watched. By the time I remembered my errand I had no idea where the tofu shop and the hospital were. I had been so fascinated by the race that it wasn't until the last runner had passed and the crowd had dispersed that I realized I was lost. I walked all over trying to retrace my steps, but it was no good. Something would seem familiar, only to turn out not to be.

Born and raised in a village, I had suddenly been thrown into a bustling town, not knowing east from west. Of course it was just a country town, with only one main street, so there was really no excuse for getting lost. But no matter where you looked, the view was the same. I couldn't get my bearings by looking at the ocean or an island or the hills. I began to cry. A woman stopped and asked, "Where are you from?" But I was crying so hard, I couldn't answer. This must have been the first time I was separated from my parents. The woman took me to a nearby police station, but I couldn't stop crying. I was even more afraid of the police than of being lost. After all, when we used to cry at home, my mother would scold us saying, "Stop that crying right now, or the police will come to get you." This was my mother's version of the old saying, "Stop crying or the *gago* will come to get you," or, "If you don't stop crying the thunder god will come and steal your belly button." In our region *gago* refers to a mysterious being, like a monster or demon. Finally I stopped crying long enough to answer their questions and explain that my mother and father were at the hospital. A policeman made a few calls and found out where I was supposed to be.

43

So, my first run-in with the police was at age six. You never forget something like that. All I had set out to do was buy one piece of tofu. As my mother and I walked back to the hospital, she pointed out the tofu shop. It wasn't more than a few doors down. Even today that street scene and the kimono pattern of the woman who helped me now and then come to mind. The fabric wasn't flashy—just a plain material. But she was such a kind person. Maybe that's why I remember her so well. After that, I would have two more close encounters with the police during my life.

At the hospital everyone was good to me. I had the run of the place and felt quite at home. Perhaps because of this positive experience early on, even today I feel at ease with strangers. Whatever the gathering, I never feel inferior. Later I left home and wandered around, but wherever I went I was blessed with kindness.

Father spent his final two weeks at the Minamata Municipal Hospital. The doctors strongly suspected that he had Minamata disease and thought it best to move him to the city hospital, where there was an isolation ward for Minamata disease patients. My father was physically spent and had lost consciousness. It was as if he were waiting to die. Only after they had exhausted all possibilities did they move him. I went back home when Father lost consciousness. Besides, they wouldn't allow family to stay at the city hospital any longer.

Although I sensed that my father was going to die, I really had no idea of what "death" might mean. I don't remember a funeral in my village until Father's death. Father passed away at the city hospital on November 27, 1959. Since we didn't have a telephone, I don't know how the hospital contacted us. At any rate, my family had already given up hope when he was transferred. By this time he was skin and bones, totally worn down by fatigue.

We all went to Minamata by boat to bring Father's body home. Father's body had already been cleaned and placed in a coffin. We had planned to take him to the home of my older sister, who had married into the nearby town of Hachiman. From there we would take him home by boat. Then a strange thing happened. The tide had gone out and our boat was stranded on the beach. It is unthinkable that fishermen would forget about the tides, but circumstances being what they were, that's what happened. There wasn't a road to my village that could be used by a hearse. We couldn't get home, so we stayed the night at my sister's and had a pre-wake. We brought him home the next day.

In this region, burial was the common practice until the mid-1960s, when it was replaced by cremation. My memories of Father's funeral are very clear. The funeral was held at our house. It was here that I first saw a camera. We all lined up and had our picture taken with the Buddhist priest. I was startled by the sound of the shutter. They took the photo twice, and you can see how surprised I look in the first one.

The day after the burial I went to the Buddhist temple with my relatives. The main building was so old that when I was running through the halls, one of the floorboards fell through. When we held the forty-ninth-day ceremony, one of my father's brothers came from Amakusa. This man looked exactly like my father. My nephew and I couldn't take our eyes off him. "Father's supposed to be dead, but he's still living," I said, and I almost called him "Dad." I remember that the adults who were in the yard watching us found this quite amusing.

My friends say that they don't remember much about what happened to them before they were of school age. When I tell them I can even remember the time I peed on Father's back, they call me a liar. But I do remember all of these things. Thinking about it now, I realize that people typically start recalling their childhood sometime in their late twenties, after they're married. But because my dear father was taken from me when I was so little, I must have made an unconscious effort to hold on to my memories of our time together.

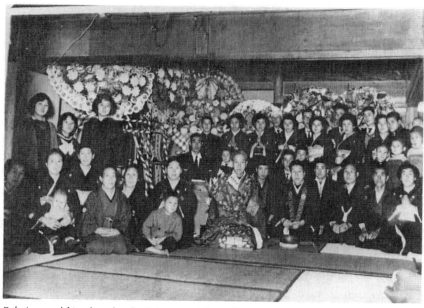

Relatives and friends gather for Fukumatsu's funeral in November 1959. Six-year-old Masato sits before his mother in the front row, peering curiously at the camera.

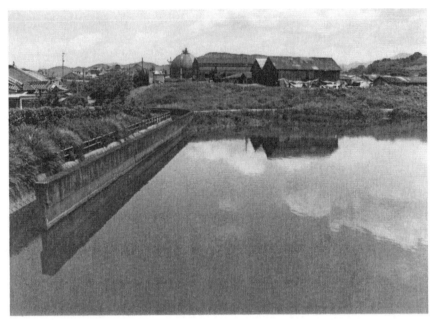

For decades Chisso's Minamata plant (background) discharged toxic wastes into an effluent canal at Hyakken Port.

Father had been so eager to see me enter elementary school. If only he could have lived another half-year. He used to tell me that he would never die before seeing that day. Even after he entered the hospital, he would deny that he might have "the strange disease" that people were talking about. I suspect that in the end he recognized that he did indeed have this new illness. It was because he realized he had it that he so forcefully denied it. I think he was trying to tell us that even if this was the strange disease, we weren't to mention it. If we did, how could we keep eating? He didn't want our family to suffer the stigma of being related to someone with this disease.

Just before my father's death in November, a fishermen's riot broke out in Minamata City. Light snow had fallen that day, and one of my brothers came home in the middle of the night saying that he'd just returned from storming the Chisso factory. Everyone sat around the fire and listened as he described how he and others had thrown bicycles and motorbikes into the canal, broken windows, destroyed desks and chairs, and chased managers out of the factory. When the managers tried to escape in motorboats, the mob chased them all around the harbor.

This turned out to be an important story for me. I had not yet seen Chisso and had no way of even imagining what the factory might look like. Adults generally referred to Chisso simply as "the Company." So, Chisso was "the Company," and "the Company" was Chisso. My older brothers said it was the Company that killed our father. However they referred to it, the idea was too abstract for me, but when my brother began describing the grounds, buildings, and canals, I began to develop a mental image. I understand now, I thought. My brothers went there to avenge my father's death.

Until my father's death, the image of Chisso had not crossed our threshold. Also, until the time of his illness, I had never handled money. These two memories became invaluable hints for understanding the nature of life around me.

Within the Circle

It was the warmth of my family that filled the void left by my father's death. My mother was with me, and my oldest brother treated me like one of his own children. Besides, my brother's wife happened to be my mother's daughter from a previous relationship, which meant that she was my sister and sister-in-law at the same time. Some might think this pretty complicated, and others might see it as a very convenient arrangement; at any rate, it was all part of my father's design. When they got married my father was already fifty-four or fifty-five—what you'd have considered an old man back in those days. He must have been thinking that he would die before my mother. As I mentioned earlier, Father was different from most people in the way he would think about life several decades down the road. As the head of a household with fifteen children, he had much to consider. There was also the fact that my mother was still in her forties. Father wanted to make sure that she would be treated well by her stepchildren.

When father was in the hospital before his death, he would struggle to draw a circle with his finger on the tatami mat. He couldn't speak, and his body trembled, but whenever one of his children came to visit he would draw a circle, as if to say, "You're to get along with each other and stay together, now, you hear?" He had been thinking about holding the family together long before he became sick. As I look back on those times, I realize now that if he hadn't planned for all of us, things wouldn't have worked out as well after his death. My father truly had amazing foresight. I grew up surrounded by all sorts of people. There were men and women, both young and old. Some were gentle, mentally handicapped folks; others were heavy drinkers, bursting with energy and always ready to pick a fight. I was a part of this group. To use my father's expression, I grew up within the circle.

In those days there wasn't a regular road all the way to the school, and even where there was a section of road we would find interesting detours. The walk home, which should have taken only an hour, would sometimes take us three

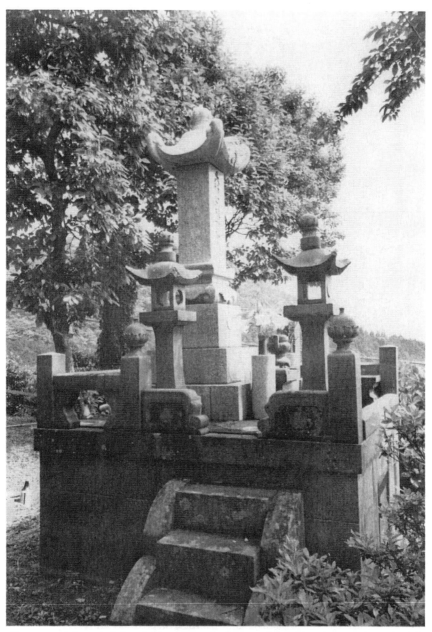

The grave of Masato's father, Fukumatsu, and other members of his clan, stands on the hill overlooking the Ogata houses, the Shiranui Sea, and the Amakusa Islands.

or four hours. As we walked through orchards we would pick fruit like persimmons, *mikan*, and loquats. The farmers would scold us when they caught us eating their fruit. On rainy days we liked to cover our heads with our school bags and wade through the shallow water along the beach. When the tide was low we would catch crabs, shrimp, and small fish hiding in the seaweed. That's what life was like for my generation. Each day brought its own adventures.

The group I hung out with included kids of all ages. The older kids could be pretty rough on us, but we learned a lot from them. We would climb plum trees and pick the green plums, burying them in the sand for a week until they turned yellow and had a nice salty taste. The older kids also taught us how to catch *mejiro*, a pretty little songbird with an olive green back, white breast, and white eye-ring. First we needed a caged *mejiro* to attract others of its kind. *Mejiro* would alight on camellia trees to suck nectar from their blossoms, so we would hang the cage high in a camellia. We would break off a branch and smear it with birdlime, spitting on our fingers all the while so the birdlime wouldn't dry and stick to our skin, and then we'd attach the branch back to the tree. Soon other *mejiro* would arrive, attracted by the calls of the caged bird. We would hide in the shadow of the trees until one alighted, and as soon as it set its feet on the lime we'd pounce on it. While we waited we would reach in our pockets for snacks of sweet potato and dried sardines. Then we would hold our breath when we saw a bird coming. Just a little bit closer, just a little closer. There! We would run out and grab it, removing the birdlime from its feet. Sometimes *mejiro* travel in flocks, and sometimes they are solitary, so there were days when we'd catch only one, or on a good day, five or six. Even after we'd caught quite a few, though, we'd select the best one, to take home as a pet, and set the others free. It's strange, but not one of us ever questioned why we should let them go. We just did it naturally.

The seventh day of the New Year was an exciting time. In our region we called the event *onibi*, or "demon fire." Our pile of branches and bamboo was as high as a house. First we used poles to make a framework, and then we tossed in dead branches on the bottom, adding greener wood toward the top. At dusk we lit the fire. Its loud, crackling sounds were said to drive away demons. We also used the fire to roast *mochi*, our New Year's rice cakes. The tip of a ten-foot bamboo pole was cut in half to hold three balls of *mochi*. A bitter orange or a *mikan* was skewered onto the tip to keep the bamboo from burning, although it may also have had a decorative function. The eating of these rice cakes was a kind of ritual, ensuring good health in the coming year. I think this event served the double function of pruning and thinning our woodlots as well as exorcising evil and misfortune. It was the children who gathered all the wood. The adults built the pile. During winter vacation, kids spent every day in the hills gathering and cutting wood. Attaching the wood to a long rope tied about their hips, they left their hands free for the trip back down. It took about ten days to two weeks to gather enough wood for the demon fire. So, our only real vacation was the first three days of the New Year.

We looked forward to the demon fire all year. It was beautiful to see the faces of friends and relatives illuminated by our giant bonfire. The flames gave our faces a rosy, healthy glow as we sat in a circle watching the blaze. Some would burn up the tips of their poles or drop their rice cakes into the fire. Others would rush off to take roasted *mochi* to their grandparents or to share some with those who were less skillful. Those were great times. Until a few years ago this custom was preserved as one of the annual events held by the primary school, but now the tradition has lapsed. In the old days we would see the flames rising from demon fires on the Amakusa Islands and other spots, and we'd think, boy, look at their fires—we have to build one just as good. Today we have lost many of the rituals that bound our communities together.

School Days

I didn't like studying. Just before I entered primary school there was an orientation day for new students. I remember that one of the teachers, Ikawa-*sensei*, asked us some questions. She showed us a triangle, a square, and a circle, and asked us to divide them each in two. Of course, you could cut the circle along any diameter, and you could divide the equilateral triangle right down the center. When it came to the square, most of the kids were dividing it in half horizontally or vertically, but I raised my hand and suggested another way. Why not cut in half diagonally? I still cherish that rare moment of praise showered on me by Ikawa-*sensei* at the start of an otherwise uninspiring school career.

Music was the only subject in which I did well. Ever since I was little I've enjoyed singing everything from children's songs to popular pieces to traditional ballads. I learned to sing by listening to my father. As for studying, I hate to sound conceited, but I was always confident that if I put my mind to my work I could do better than anyone. But from the time I was small, I was told by my older brothers and everyone else that studying was not for me. "Out at sea you want to catch fish, not letters," they would say. I remember wishing in the fifth or sixth grade that I could go on to high school. But my family said I could only complete the compulsory education program, which just took me through junior high. If I had been told that I could continue, I'm sure I would have studied.

Perhaps this wasn't so bad, though, because I learned at an early age that book learning wasn't everything. Life had more important things to teach. I began going out on a fishing boat with my father when I could barely walk, and while I was in primary school I often joined my older brothers. The work was tough, but we had fun. My father went through only the second year of primary school, and my brothers spent more time fishing than attending class. Observing them, I realized that a person could make a living without going to school. Besides, it was more fun to work with living things.

After my father died and I entered primary school, I began to rebel against my mother. For example, I remember this incident. You have to buy a new uniform for the entrance ceremony to primary or middle school. My mother let me wear the new uniform only on the day of the ceremony itself; it would be a shame if it got dirty, she said. All of the other children wore their new uniform, while I wore shabby old clothes. I was ashamed and hated her for treating me like this. But at other times, she would spoil me to an extreme. On Parents' Day she came to school to observe our class. While all the other kids had young parents, my mother had already turned fifty. Both her features and clothing looked old. In her blind devotion, she had eyes only for me, and when she opened her mouth, it was obvious that she had no idea of my class standing. I begged her not to visit the school again.

After I entered middle school, my mother kept nagging at me to become a carpenter or a plasterer. But from the time my father died my brothers told me to become a fisherman, and that was my own wish all along. One reason my mother tried to head me toward another profession was that she had been raised in a farming family. "Beggars can escape bad weather under a bridge or in a Shinto shrine, but fishermen have to go out to sea even when it's raining and blowing. They're lowlier than beggars," my mother would say. She would also repeat a tale about a beggar's child who wouldn't stop crying. The little girl's mother scolded her, saying, "If you don't stop crying we'll marry you off to a fisherman!" Such was the pitiful status of a fisherman.

In primary school they had us write compositions. On Father's Day we were told to return the next day with an essay about our dads. I didn't want to, so I turned in a blank piece of paper. The teacher got mad, so I asked, "How can I write about someone who isn't here?" He was taken aback and responded, "Well, write about your mother, then." "That wasn't the assignment," I replied. There were two other kids in the class who didn't have fathers, but the teacher was too insensitive to think about it. Those two wrote essays on some other theme.

In the upper level of primary school, we read about Minamata disease in one of our textbooks. Our teachers mentioned the disease in class but showed no sensitivity toward children like me whose families had been directly affected. I tried to endure those moments in silence. The teacher summarily dismissed the topic, saying, "A company called Chisso dumped some toxic waste, and many people were killed." When I reminded him that I had lost my father to Minamata disease, he turned pale. Since teachers often visited the homes of their pupils, he should have known about my family.

The students could be cruel as well. From about the third grade, kids began ridiculing me. After picking a fight with me, they would sneer in front of the others, "His father died of Minamata disease." On the way to and from school I would sometimes pass housewives who would start gossiping behind my back, "That's the son of Fukumatsu-*san*, who died of the strange disease." They made me so angry. Originally Chisso had been known as a manufacturer of chemical fertilizers. Whenever I came across one of Chisso's bags in the fields, I would kick it angrily.

Fighting among school kids was an everyday occurrence. Verbal sparring was rare; we usually resorted to brute force. But by the time we entered middle school, we were better friends with those we had fought than with the other kids. I never fought with the more serious, studious kids, but I never made friends with them, either. Fights often occurred between kids of different villages, so those belonging to the same hamlet would hang together, even though their ages might differ a lot. When trouble started, neighborhood kids would draw together. At a signal from the older kids, we'd begin throwing stones. The strange thing is that I don't recall anyone ever being so seriously injured that he had to go to the hospital. We must have fought so often that we knew how to do it without really hurting each other.

It was not until I reached the fourth or fifth grade that I began to realize that I might be physically inferior to the average kid my age. I slowly learned that other kids didn't have the dizzy spells I frequently experienced. I would become fatigued more easily than others. I was the worst stone-thrower among my friends. I began to wonder why I was like this, but it did not occur to me that these were all initial symptoms of Minamata disease. During my middle-school years I started to experience numbness in my hands, legs, and feet, and around my mouth. The numbness became worse when I was sick or tired. The symptoms were worst from late spring to the rainy season in early summer. Even then I had no idea that the problem was there to stay. To me, Minamata disease was something more serious and drastic, as it had been for my father, and for my nephew and niece, born with congenital Minamata disease. It was not until the early 1970s that I understood clearly that I was one of the many Minamata disease sufferers. Each sufferer had slightly different symptoms, reflecting the patient's degree of exposure and personal health.

A Family Ordeal

In the 1960s, young people abandoned our region in droves to search for employment in urban centers. As televisions and refrigerators flowed in, the labor force flowed out. My family managed to keep fishing even after Father's death, but our need for cash increased. The children in school needed books and other supplies, and the farm required fertilizer and new machinery and tools. It must have been when I was in primary school that instant ramen first appeared. Until fast foods became popular, we had been delighted just to find a fried egg in our lunch boxes.

As I grew up, I became keenly interested in politics. Although my grades were low, I doubt that any of my classmates expressed as great an interest in public affairs. I even learned the names and faces of all the cabinet members. I felt that if the government had been run properly, something as horrible as the Minamata disease incident would never have occurred. The conservative Liberal Democratic Party was in power. Therefore, emotionally I leaned toward the socialist and communist opposition parties. This was when Prime Minister Sato Eisaku was in power. There was much fighting between intra-party factions, and politicians were held in general distrust. Even though I was just a child, I wished that I could turn the world around. I intuitively felt that it was not Chisso by itself but society as a whole—the system that dictated the actions of a company like Chisso—that was wrong. I understood full well that the ruling party focused its attention on the growth of such large corporations. This focus is what I wanted to change.

In 1968 the government officially recognized Minamata disease as a condition caused by industrial pollution, and the next year victims filed a class-action suit against the government. Before the suit was filed, my family was faced with the decision of whether or not to participate as plaintiffs. At that time there was only one victims' organization, but it was already divided between those who wanted to file suit and those who didn't. Those who opposed the suit worried that the costs would be so high they would jeopardize the family assets, and they were concerned about alienating themselves from their neighbors. The same things concerned my brothers and sisters when they got together to talk about what role our family should play. This happened right after I graduated from middle school. I was in favor of going to court, but I was the only one in my family who felt this way.

In 1959, ten years before this civil suit was filed, Chisso had offered the victims what was called a "sympathy payment" contract. Gifts of money to the victims, the company hoped, would enable it to settle the affair once and for all. The terms were outrageous, enabling the company, for example, to compensate for the death of one adult with three hundred thousand yen ($833, at 360 yen to the dollar). The contract contained a clause that said that even if the source of Minamata disease were to be linked to Chisso, victims would agree not to demand further compensation. I think everyone felt constrained by this agreement. (Later, the contract was declared invalid and thrown out by the court as a violation of basic ethical standards.) But I just couldn't swallow these terms, so I begged my brothers not to feel bound by such a paltry sum of money, and to take a stand in court. In the end, however, my family didn't join the suit. "We might lose everything we've got," said my brothers. "It's easier to run with the tide."

It wasn't that someone influenced me to promote the lawsuit. I reached this decision on my own. Surely there was no way the victims could lose. I also wanted to strike back at Chisso and to clarify the company's responsibility. I didn't know that I too was affected by mercury poisoning. I didn't know a thing about trials. But I did know that I had to do something to avenge my father's death, for he was a man I had loved and respected above all others.

During the same year that my father passed away, one of my nieces, Hitomi, was born with Minamata disease. Her body was deformed, and for the longest time she couldn't hold up her head. She would cry all night. Even if we held her, changed her diapers, or gave her milk, she wouldn't stop crying. Life must be really hard for her, I felt. My nephew Tatsuzumi is also a victim of congenital Minamata disease. Since we all ate the same fish, there isn't one of us that wasn't affected to some extent by the poison. A survey was conducted in 1960 of the mercury content in the hair of local residents. My hair contained about 182 parts per million (ppm) of mercury. Hitomi's four-year-old brother—not a congenital victim—registered 224 ppm, and three-month-old Hitomi, 33.5 ppm. The mercury content in the hair of a healthy Japanese person at that time averaged one to five ppm. Eventually ten members of the Ogata family were officially recognized as Minamata disease victims: my parents and eight of my brothers, sisters, and their children.

After Father died, Minamata disease became so prevalent in my family that people began to say it must be a genetic problem. In a remote village like ours, this type of gossip might well have been the product of some long-smoldering envy of a well-established family. "The Ogata family was once so prosperous," they would begin. Other men in our village had died in much the same way that my father had, but no one was willing to trace the causes of their deaths to Minamata disease. If they had admitted the roots of the problem, as my family had, they in turn would have become the object of village gossip. Some rumors would hold that the disease was genetic, and some would say it was infectious. Through these rumors Minamata disease became a social stigma, which made it difficult for young people to find marriage partners or employment. If families accepted compensation for death or illness, they would be accused of taking Chisso's dirty money. So, families who lost a loved one to Minamata disease would attribute the death to any number of other afflictions. Even the victims themselves must have wanted to believe that they had anything but Minamata disease.

This was the general atmosphere until the first judicial decision was reached. However, as the case progressed and the issue was covered on television and in the press, Chisso's responsibility became a topic of public discussion. As the disease became more socially acceptable, the number of victims applying for certification increased. But even so, they would try to apply in such a way that none of their neighbors knew about it. There was no way that our family could hide its victims from the outside world, but the same doubts and social stigmas cast a shadow over our lives. No one wanted to talk about it. Of course, there wasn't anything positive to say, but I thought it was essential to deal with our situation. My mother and brothers would often tell me that nothing we said about Minamata disease could bring my father back to life, so there was no point in discussing it.

My niece Hitomi, with congenital Minamata disease, is getting by, although her limbs are unsteady. As part of her physical therapy at a residential care facility she weaves rushes into mats. She's a tough girl. Some years ago a crew from NHK television came by wanting to film a scene of me talking with Hitomi. I was skeptical as to whether Hitomi would accept such a proposition, but to my surprise, she was quite willing. She said she had no intention of remaining hidden. "Don't you hate Chisso?" I asked. "No," she answered. "Because I'd rather focus on how I'm going to live in the future than on what happened in the past." I must say that among the younger victims there is a tendency to develop a dependent mentality. Perhaps it's because the people helping them out are overly careful and attentive. Anybody can talk about how bad Minamata disease is and how bad Chisso is, but very few can talk about their own lives. Hitomi, however, is determined to live without allowing Minamata disease to define who she is and will be. Against her parents' wishes she entered a girls' high school in Kumamoto and lived in the dormitory for three years. She's a determined young woman, all right, and I admire her.

As I was growing up, my nephew and niece were like brother and sister to me. Living with the handicapped was a part of my life, and I wanted to do anything I could to protect them from the outside world. In this I was probably influenced a great deal by my father. Although I haven't been able to match my father's financial success, it makes me happy that lately my sisters have been saying that I'm becoming more and more like him.

Over the years my family learned to live with the fate of Minamata disease. But even so, I would ask myself as a child, why it was that this disease was concentrated so heavily in one family? We were different from other afflicted people, though, in that we knew exactly who was responsible and had some outlet for our anger. In fact, I wanted to avenge what they had done to us. But anger and hatred could not erase the question, "Why us?"

Diseases caused by industrial pollution are often viewed simply as tragedies for the victims. But as a Minamata disease patient, I can now say that while this disease is a tragedy, we can also look at it as an ordeal to be overcome. In this sense, Minamata disease victims are no different than other handicapped people. If we define ourselves as victims, we won't get anywhere. Only when we embrace Minamata disease as a condition with which we live will we be able to keep moving forward.

Leaving Home

After I graduated from junior high, I worked for my family for one year. Then, at age sixteen, I left home. It was a beautiful day when I walked to the town of Sashiki, carrying a single bag. This was right about the time when the express bus *Hayabusa* had started the run to Kumamoto City, the capital and largest city in our prefecture. I believe the fare was 360 yen (one dollar) from the Sashiki train station to Kumamoto. I had fifteen thousand yen on me. On the way to the bus stop I ran into a neighbor, Ikeda-*san*. I wasn't dressed up, but he seemed to sense that I was going somewhere. He asked where I was headed; I didn't know how to answer but somehow I skirted around the question. All the way to the station I had kept asking myself if I shouldn't go back home, and running into Ikeda-*san* reinforced my doubts. If I were to go back right away, no one would even know I was missing. It's pretty interesting, but when you get to a major crossroads like this in your life, you have any number of chances to change your mind. While I was still thinking about leaving, and even after I had taken off, I had many opportunities to reverse course.

I'd been thinking of leaving home for six months. One reason was that the fishing industry was in decline. For another thing, my brother, who had become the family head, was a violent alcoholic. When he was sober he was a great guy, but once he was drunk nobody could touch him. It got to the point that he would become violent about twice a week. He never mistreated me, but he used to break things and beat his own family. I couldn't take it any longer. I had been witness to this behavior since I was little, but I'd decided in my own heart that I would stay at home and work—and I did my very best to help him. But my brother didn't change. Why couldn't he understand what he was doing? In desperation, I went to talk to my oldest sister, but there was nothing we could do. It was around that time that I began to think of leaving home.

I didn't entertain any feelings of guilt for leaving my brother's house. Rather, it was my brother who must have felt guilty for making me want to leave. But if you ask whether I was angry with him or hated him, I truly didn't. I knew very well how hard life was for him. He was just in his twenties when Father died, and from that moment he had to bear all responsibility for our family affairs. After Father's death, his employees gradually acquired their own boats and began to leave. Our fishing operation grew smaller and smaller. People would compare my brother's performance with Father's. All of these things must have contributed to my brother's alcoholism. About a year after I left home, my brother suffered a heart attack in the middle of the night and passed away.

Of course I realized that my family would worry about me when I left home, but what concerned me most was whether I could overcome the mag-netism of this place—my village, the land, and the sea. Until then, this had been my whole universe. There was nothing I could rely on once I left. No matter where I would go in the village, I knew that any family would have put me up, even for a week or two. But now I was entering an unknown world. I didn't know anyone. I didn't know where to go. I didn't have much money. So this is what it's like to leave everything you know and love, I thought.

One of my main reasons for leaving home was that I wanted to prove myself; I wanted to become a success. Also, like my brother, I was tired of trying to live up to my father's image. Even now my cousins will say things like, "Look what your father accomplished in just one generation, while you . . ." I was probably trying to escape these critical comparisons. I had a lot of things to run away from, but I hadn't given any thought to where I was running or what I might like to do. My only plan was to go to Osaka, because most young folks who left this area in search of work migrated to that big metropolitan center.

Even after getting on the bus, I still thought about returning, but as it sped on toward Kumamoto, my doubts grew weaker with each passing mile. I can't say that I was looking straight into the future, but there was certainly no going back. When I got off the bus at a huge terminal in Kumamoto City I was already lost. So I decided to just walk around and familiarize myself with the town. As I walked, I kept an eye out for help-wanted signs. I began to cover the city, block by block. Eventually I found a welder's shop, and I went in to ask if they could hire me. But because I'd been a fisherman, my face was dark from the sun. On top of that, I was dressed like a country bumpkin and was carrying a bag—a sure runaway. Everywhere I stopped, the people just shooed me out, without even talking to me. Just so I could sit down somewhere, I went to a movie theater. They were playing a pornographic film. I could hardly believe what I was seeing. I had never seen anything like that before.

When I stepped out of the theater it was already dark. I remember buying some pastries to curb my hunger. Although I had a little money, I knew that if I stayed at an inn I'd be broke in no time. So, I decided to sleep on a bench next to a bus stop. It was the coldest time of winter. I curled up and went to sleep. It must have been around three or 3:30 in the morning when someone woke me up, saying, "Hey, hey you." It was a man who looked a little over twenty years old. "What the hell are you doing here?" he asked. But his voice showed such concern that I confessed I had run away from home. He introduced himself as Tanaka. After we'd talked a bit, he invited me to stay at his place. Just in front of the bus stop was a Turkish bath called the "Mona Lisa." That's where Tanaka's girlfriend worked. In fact, Tanaka was her pimp, and he was there to pick her up as she finished her shift. Soon I was riding in a cab with this couple and found myself at a cheap, rundown apartment house near Suizenji Station.

Tanaka's floor was divided into six small rooms, each four and a half tatami mats in size. Each room was a separate apartment, with a sink and a closet. All shared one communal toilet. As we sat in the little room I looked around and realized that the only furniture was a small tea table. There was nothing else to do but go to bed. Although I was very tired, I couldn't sleep a wink. Fortunately they had two sets of futons, but they were embracing right next to me. I'd never seen anyone do that. At my house I had always slept in a large room; in fact, our spacious country house didn't even have a room this small. What made it worse was that I could hear voices in the neighboring rooms and the creaking of footsteps down the hall. I couldn't believe that anyone could live this way.

Finally, around seven o'clock, the sun came up, so I hurried out to the toilet, but instead of going back to the room I decided to explore the neighborhood. Getting up early and working was my regular routine, and besides, I needed some exercise. Apparently when Tanaka and his girlfriend awakened to find me gone, they were pretty upset. They couldn't imagine anyone wanting to get up that early and thought I must have robbed them and taken off. But they soon noticed that I'd left my bag and that nothing of theirs was missing, so they became concerned and went out to look for me. "We thought you'd ripped us off," Tanaka told me later. "What on earth would I find to steal?" I returned. As far as I could see, the girlfriend's earnings at the Turkish bath was their only income, and they were living day to day. I gave up my plan to go to Osaka and ended up staying with this couple in Kumamoto City.

I wanted to find a job, so I went to an employment agency, but they weren't very helpful. The main problem was that I didn't have a guarantor, as required of a teenager seeking a job, and I hadn't filed a change of residency form. With Tanaka's help, though, a week later I found a job with a trucking company as a driver's assistant. I worked hard for this company for about six months. I stayed with Tanaka the whole time, but his four-and-a-half-mat room was really too small for three people, so we moved into a six-mat room downstairs. Until the first payday I was dependent on Tanaka—or, I should say, his girlfriend. But even after I began to receive a salary, life wasn't that easy. After three months or so my monthly pay went up to thirty thousand yen (eighty-three dollars), of which I gave Tanaka ten thousand, and I paid the company ten thousand for meals. This left me with ten thousand yen for myself. I was barely hanging on.

It wasn't that Tanaka had told me to get a job. Rather, it seems that he wanted me to become his gangster protégé. As one month passed and then two, he grew quite fond of me. He even took me to his home village to visit his family. His parents farmed in a rural area of northern Kumamoto Prefecture. I helped them out in the busy rice-planting season, and soon his family also became attached to me. In this way I began to meet people through Tanaka, and I felt happy about the network of friends I was developing. Among these acquaintances were people who worked for the Turkish bath and some of Tanaka's shady counterparts.

This new life was kind of like a school—a place where I learned about drinking, women, and gambling. One day Tanaka asked me, "Have you ever been with a woman?" When I said I hadn't, he replied, "I'm going to take you somewhere." He took me to another Turkish bath. As he paid one of the women, he said, "This kid don't know nothin'. Teach him a few things." And he left. I was shocked. In those days Turkish baths weren't necessarily places where you could have sex. Only more limited sexual contact was allowed. The bath owners were careful not to go beyond the limits of the law, and the women were supposed to keep on their underwear as they bathed the men. But of course this was my first time, and I didn't know any of these things. "No thanks," I said, and started to leave. "There's no need to be shy," the woman said in a kind voice. "I'll show you what to do." As I followed her down the corridor, the garish red and blue lights may have disguised my embarrassment, but when we walked into a room I couldn't bring myself to undress. "Just slip them off," she urged, helping me off with my clothes and leaving me naked. We didn't exactly have sex, but it was close enough. I had never been touched like that before. Regardless of my confusion, my young body acted almost independently. I had never imagined it would feel so good.

I put everything into my job. I would arrive thirty minutes before my shift began and wash our truck. Everyone liked me. As a trucker's assistant my main job was to load and unload cement bags, rice, and furniture. In our busy season I would move up to five households a day, carrying furniture up and down many flights of stairs with the help of the driver. Slowly I began to realize that city people were always trying to figure out a way to shirk hard work. But I always threw myself into a task wholeheartedly, so all the drivers would compete to work with me. This is how, after just three months, I managed to get promoted from a temporary to a full-time position and received a raise of fifty yen per day.

A mover's job is interesting, because you can see how people live. Some families were all ready when we arrived, while others didn't even begin packing until we got there. I could also figure out the nature of a couple's relationship by listening to them talk. I remember one incident in particular. We were delivering furniture to a shabby little house. Usually people will move to a better place than they were before, but this was the opposite. We were supposed to be paid cash on delivery, but the husband said he would send it later. They looked so poor that we decided to leave without demanding the money. When we got back to the office and explained the situation to the manager, he was furious and sent us back to demand payment. But the husband told us that he was broke. I realized that they must have had to move for failure to pay rent at their previous place. I felt sorry for the man and decided to have the company deduct the charge from my salary. When we showed up at the office again without payment, the boss was even angrier. I wanted to ask him how you could extract money from someone who doesn't have any, but instead I just told him to take it out of my wages. The boss didn't say any more about it. Looking at the way all these different people lived and behaved was to contribute a great deal to my understanding of life.

A Compass Restored

One day while I was sitting in our truck waiting for the light to change, we were hit from behind. This put me in the hospital for two weeks with a swollen neck. After a month I had recovered completely, but Tanaka said, "We could use this to make money, so keep on going to the hospital." I felt bad about it, but I did what Tanaka told me. It was like magic. I could play every day, and more money poured in than when I had been working. Now that I had both money and time, it was natural that Tanaka's lifestyle began to brush off on me. I would go with him to *pachinko* parlors. By then Tanaka and I were like brothers. It wasn't that I enjoyed this kind of lifestyle. I had never had any interest in *pachinko*, but Tanaka was an inveterate gambler. Because he couldn't control himself, he would put me in charge of his wallet. When he was on a losing streak, I refused to give him any more money. There were times when I'd even start lecturing him, "Why don't you think about your father and your younger sisters once in a while!" Even then Tanaka never got mad. He was always nice to me.

Tanaka's friends belonged to one of Kumamoto's right-wing political organizations, which was also a front for criminal *yakuza* operations. I started to hang out there and became friendly with many of the people. Sometimes I even stayed over and began to learn what they were about. I found that they were involved in selling amphetamines, loan sharking, and fraud. One of their tricks was to open luxurious jewelry stores. In their initial dealings with wholesalers, their checks would be good. But once they established their credit, they would place a large order for jewelry and then disappear overnight with the goods. They would work as a team, with specialists in this type of operation. These guys would always disappear on a Friday, so it wouldn't be noticed that they were gone until Monday.

I tried amphetamines about five times. They made me feel really good, but coming down was horrible. A terrible fatigue would sweep over me. The senior gangsters told us not to use these drugs—they knew very well what would happen to us in the end. Despite what these men did for a living, they all seemed pretty nice to me. They wouldn't bother people in the street. I'm not saying every criminal is like that; maybe those I met were exceptions. But as for me, I must admit that I lost my soul. Without knowing it, I was being assimilated into an underworld of gamblers, drug dealers, and petty thieves. My political interests, anger at society, and bitterness toward Chisso were being overshadowed by my new life.

After a while I, too, became a member of this right-wing organization. Almost by osmosis I came to adopt their political views. Their two main political slogans were "Crush the All-Japan Teachers' Union" and "Reclaim the Northern Islands from the Soviet Union." But as I said, their political propaganda was a front for criminal activity, and the members didn't really take these issues very seriously. I never saw them studying anything. Once I asked them, "Why *do* we have to support the Emperor, anyway?" They were visibly shaken, but I continued, "Wouldn't we get along fine without him?" After a long silence, one guy asked me, "Are you Red?" I didn't see why they were so upset. It seemed like a very natural and innocent question to me.

I understand now that those guys never truly believed what they were saying. They were just mouthing catchphrases, because they thought it was the thing to do. Their political activism was only meant to remind the world of their existence. The young people they recruited couldn't have cared less about such issues as the Teachers' Union or the dispute about the northern islands. Even I didn't apply much logic to my thinking. This was the sort of organization that attracted people who were incapable of logical reasoning. Most of the recruits were from poor, dysfunctional families. When leftist political organizations went about recruiting new members, they would begin by testing their political convictions. But the right-wingers didn't seem to care about a person's politics. They would always start out, "You look like you're broke. Let's go get a bite to eat together—my treat." If the left wing ever learned this approach from the right wing, they might have a larger organization.

One day in early September, in my second year away from home, I happened to see a huge billboard as I was walking in front of Kumamoto University. It was a political announcement urging students to join a rally to stop the Self-Defense Forces from being dispatched to Okinawa. About that time there was a meeting of right-wing organizations in the city, and I made a proposal. I told them about the announcement at the university and asked them if we were going to do something about it. My suggestion probably reminded them of what their political goals were supposed to be. They decided to confront the left-wing students.

Several hundred students held a demonstration and marched from Kumamoto University to the Shimizu Self-Defense Force base, where we were waiting. The students had their faces covered with masks and were wearing helmets. There were about thirty of us, wearing khaki combat uniforms and flying a flag from a jeep. We had all been told not to make a move until we received orders. At the base, armed members of the Self-Defense Force were guarding the gate. Just in front of them stood the riot police, and curious bystanders lined the sidewalks. There must have been over two thousand people, and the air was thick with tension. But after what seemed to me hours of students chanting meaningless slogans and marching around, it became apparent to me that there wasn't going to be any kind of physical confrontation.

When the student demonstrators began to withdraw, I charged toward them. I felt that if I let them go like this, the whole event would have been meaningless. All the words and gestures would have been wasted, and I didn't want to be part of such an empty ceremony. I couldn't wait any longer for an order. I started out empty-handed but grabbed a piece of fallen lumber along the way and began to beat the students with it. Within seconds the riot police were after me, and I was caught. Taking advantage of my helplessness, the students seized the opportunity to spear me with their bamboo flagpoles. I was terrified as the sharp spears closed in. Even after I was dragged into the police van, the students tried to get at me through the windows.

To my surprise, the police already knew my name and address. It was clear that they had been checking up on me. I was detained at the police station for several days. At first I felt proud of taking action that I knew full well might lead to my arrest. I was also proud of the fact that I refused to speak of my association with the political organization. I knew that those who talked didn't even garner the respect of the police. I was eventually sent to a juvenile correction center, where I was locked up for six weeks. I shouldn't have been detained that long, because I was a first offender and hadn't committed a major crime. The reason they kept me there was that I wouldn't cooperate with the police and confess to anything.

While I was at the correction center, a counselor spent some time talking with me. "You seem to be proud of having joined a right-wing organization," he said, "but didn't your father die of Minamata disease? Do you know what these right-wing groups really represent?" He told me that Minamata disease patients holding a protest demonstration at Chisso's headquarters in Tokyo had been attacked by a group of right-wing thugs hired by the company. I didn't know how to respond. For the first time in my life, I found myself at a loss for words. Then the counselor added, "You don't belong in a place like this. Go back to your village." It was true. I had felt from the start that I was really quite different from the guys I was hanging out with. Regional dialect kept creeping into my speech; my face was black from working in the sun;

even my features seemed different. I was a stranger. Although I had become involved in lots of questionable activities, I was not committed to this way of life. Eventually the correction center requested that some of my family come to talk to me. They begged me to come home. At first I was too embarrassed to return. I had run away with the dream of becoming a success. But in actuality I had become a failure and ended up in jail. I had no idea how I would face my family and village again. But finally I was persuaded, and I agreed to go home.

After I left the correction center I spent three days making the rounds of friends and acquaintances to thank them for their kindness to me and explain why I was leaving. My family, who had come to take me home, must have been pretty worried about giving me three more days in which I might become ensnared again by the same bad influences. The gangster world is known for its reluctance to let people go. I thought I might even have to cut off my little finger as the price for my freedom. But my decision to leave was firm, and I knew it was important for me to be courteous to those who had taken me in and helped me. Going from one person to the next, I expressed my gratitude. They were all aware of the fact that I had not talked to the police, and this probably made it a lot easier for me to leave. Also, I discovered that they respected me for making an independent decision to attack the student demonstrators. I guess they saw this as a contribution to their cause. It turned out to have been good publicity for the organization.

The most difficult part was saying good-bye to Tanaka. By then we were as close as real brothers, and he didn't want to let me go. During the three days I was making my rounds, he tried to convince me to stay. But I simply told him, "This is my decision, and I'm going to stick by it. I'm going home."

Looking back, I'm amazed at how much I learned during those two years away from home. I met so many different people. Although I saw some of the weakness and ugliness of human nature, I still feel fortunate to have been surrounded by those I met. They were all good to me, and I know I was lucky to have been able to leave without too much difficulty. I wonder what sort of life I would be leading now if I had stayed? I'm quite certain that it would have been morally bankrupt, and I never would have rediscovered my soul.

Part Two

常世の舟

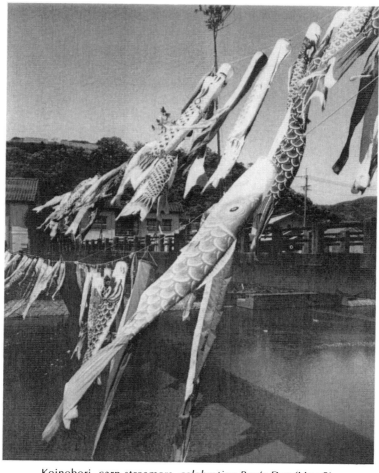

Koinobori, *carp streamers, celebrating Boy's Day (May 5),*
along Sashiki River

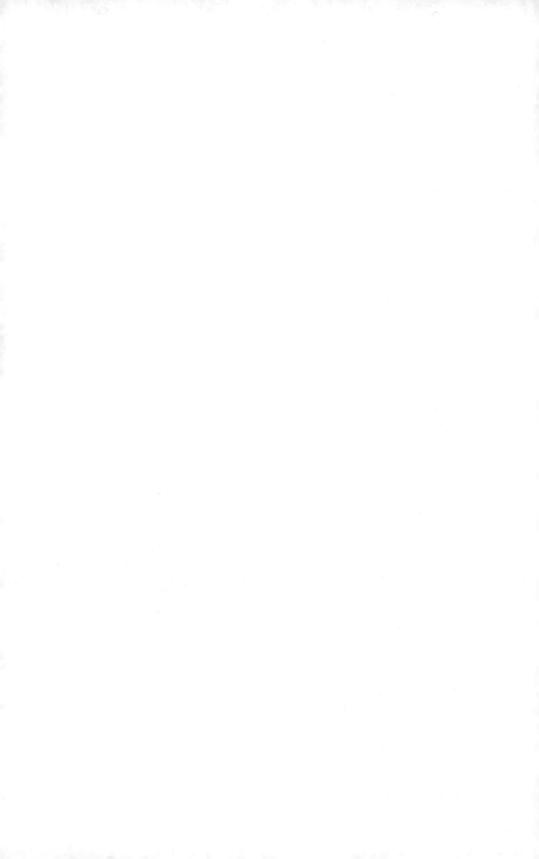

Rising Tides

As I headed home, I was filled with apprehension. I had left the village with high hopes, yet I was returning with nothing. Surely the villagers would have learned about the kind of life I had been leading. It wouldn't be easy to regain their acceptance. I would probably have to endure their criticism and ridicule. But I had made up my mind that this would be a fresh start. No matter what happened, I would give it at least six months. If things didn't get better, I would hold out a little longer. That's what I decided.

As I had expected, the villagers treated me coldly. Even my brothers, sisters, and other relatives let me know, in their attitudes if not in their words, that I was a disgrace to the family. It was painful. In three or four months, though, their stance softened, and by the time six months had passed they were actually warming to me.

For a year and a half after my return I lived with one of my sisters and her husband in the village, helping out with their fishing operation. But I didn't want to be an assistant forever, so I decided to strike out on my own. My family agreed to finance the construction of a ten-meter fishing boat for two of my nephews and me. This boat belonged to the last generation of wooden fishing vessels built by traditional methods. The three of us went up to the mountains with the boat builder to select a suitable tree. A Japanese cedar, *sugi*, about two hundred years old is ideal for the main body of a boat. When the tree was cut we performed a ritual ceremony. The lumberjack placed offerings of salt and rice under the cedar, and we prayed to the spirits of the forest.

We named our boat *Wakashio*, "Young Tide," which refers to the rising tides between neap tide and spring tide. We picked this name as a symbol of our youth and as a prayer for our success—three young men on the verge of a bright and prosperous future. In spite of our hopes and prayers, however, our boat was not destined to turn the tide of our coastal fishing culture.

Soon after our boat was built, the third outbreak of Minamata disease was reported in the Ariake Sea and in Tokuyama Bay.[1] Consumers nationwide panicked over the possibility of mercury poisoning, and fish prices plummeted. Since Chisso had stopped using mercury around 1967, there shouldn't have been any more poisoned fish in our region, except in Minamata Bay. But as soon as consumers heard the words "mercury poisoning," they associated it with Minamata and refused to buy fish from us. What else could we do to make a living? We had grown up with fish.

As I look back on my life, I can see that this third outbreak of Minamata disease formed a strong undercurrent, directing my future. In the aftermath of the latest mercury poisoning panic, the Shiranui Sea Fishermen's Union once again demanded compensation from Chisso and blockaded the factory. Until this time Chisso had not provided compensation to any group other than the Minamata Fishermen's Association of Minamata City. The Shiranui Fishermen's Union was demanding an enormous sum—something like fifteen billion yen. In July all the boats affiliated with the union converged to protest against Chisso. Several boats from my hometown, Meshima, were among the protesters. My neighbors and I got in my boat and headed out, with a military march blaring out over the loudspeakers. Although we hadn't meant to, we arrived ahead of everyone else. It felt good to be in the lead— like a naval commander directing a fleet. As we entered Minamata Bay and started to turn, all the other boats followed us.

When we reached port, we held a rally on shore. Then we marched to the front gates of Chisso. This was the beginning of a land and sea blockade, as well as picketing campaign, that was to last two months. Each fishermen's association was in charge of a particular site, and we worked in three-day shifts. My association was in charge of the main gate. Others blockaded Umedo Port, the entryway for raw materials shipped to Chisso, as well as the small feeder lines to the trunk line of the Kumamoto Railway. We set up a tent at the main entrance with an opening just wide enough to admit one person at a time, and we didn't let any materials through. This is how I found myself standing for the first time in front of Chisso, the company I had known from early childhood to be my family's greatest enemy.

As it turned out, my boat *Wakashio* saw its greatest use in the protest movement. By this time our family fishing business was in decline. Most fishermen in the region had already switched to *tai* (red snapper) farming. Small boats still fished the bay, but you would seldom see a large boat like ours. My older nephew moved into agriculture, working in the rice fields and tending *mikan* orchards. Eventually my younger nephew, from the main house, also left to become apprenticed to a carpenter. As I grew increasingly involved with the movement, I too spent less and less time fishing.

The year of our protest, 1973, was significant for another reason. While the third outbreak of Minamata disease was making national news, the courts

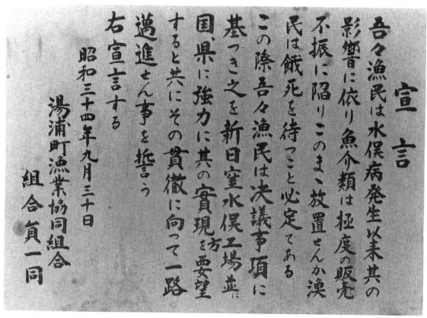

宣言

吾々漁民は水俣病発生以来其の影響に依り魚介類は極度の販売不振に陥りこのまゝ放置せんか漁民は餓死を待つこと必定である

この際吾々漁民は決議事項に基づき之を新日窒水俣工場並に国、県に強力に其の実現を要望するとと共にその貫徹に向って一路邁進せん事を誓う

右宣言する

昭和三十四年九月三十日

湯浦町漁業協同組合

組合員一同

A manifesto on the signboard by the fishermen's union of Yunoura on September 30, 1959, swears uncompromising struggle against Chisso, Kumamoto Prefecture, and the state (Soshisha exhibit).

handed down a decision in the first Minamata disease lawsuit. The government had officially acknowledged in 1968 that Minamata disease was the result of industrial pollution; the following year, a victims' group filed a lawsuit. After four years of court proceedings, the victims won their case, and the court ruled that Chisso would be required to enter a compensation agreement. After this we shifted our focus to the problem of obtaining recognition of patients not yet certified as Minamata disease victims. Chisso's social responsibility toward the victims had at last been publicly affirmed, an important turning point for the patients. Patients other than the plaintiffs were brought together by the necessity to apply for certification, and in 1974 a new organization was formed, the Minamata Disease Certification Applicants' Council. The formation of the council marked a new stage in our struggle.

The decisive turning point for me, however, was my exposure to the young supporters who had begun to flood in from outside. In the summer of 1973 four student radicals who wanted to support the Minamata disease movement came to my village. There were three men and one woman. They rented a house near mine and named it "China Boat Cottage," after a famous rock just offshore. I spent a lot of time there. But the village as a whole was leery of their presence, and they weren't even allowed to become involved with the village youth association. It's not surprising that the village held them in suspicion; after all, they were total strangers who had suddenly dropped in our midst. My reaction was quite the opposite. These strangers aroused my curiosity. Who were they, and what were they thinking? I managed to get them into the youth association by telling the villagers that I would serve as guarantor. Some villagers still shied away from the idea, but I insisted, saying, "Don't worry, I'll take full responsibility for them." Responsibility? And just what was I going to do? Looking back on it now, I have to laugh.

I was unrelenting in my attempts to get to know the students. I stopped by constantly with gifts of *shochu* and fish, sometimes keeping them up talking until two or three in the morning; if they didn't watch out, I'd be there all night. I was determined to learn something about these outsiders of my own generation. It was easy to understand how someone like me would feel anger and hatred toward Chisso, the company responsible for my father's death, but how could these outsiders claim to share my emotions? How could they act without any personal motives? Was it really possible for outsiders to take up a cause and make it their own? These questions burned in my mind.

I have to admit that I was also just plain curious. This was my first opportunity to hang out with university students. Contrary to my image of the serious intellectual, these students were quite down to earth. We had a great time playing *shogi* together. They led the simplest of lifestyles. Apparently all of their clothes and food had been donated by friends and supporters. Pictures of Marx, Lenin, and Mao decorated their walls. I once asked them, "Who *are* these old men?" "You don't know?" they replied in amazement. Of course, I recognized the names, but I'd never seen the faces. At any rate, the students never said much about these men or their own political ideologies.

When it came to Chisso Company and the Minamata disease incident, however, the students knew far more than I did. I flooded them with questions. It became clear that apart from my well-directed anger against Chisso, I was pretty ignorant about the complexity of the issues. I didn't know anything about the role of politics, government administration, and the Japanese state in the Minamata disease incident. I didn't understand anything about the chemical and biological aspects of mercury poisoning, or its medical implications. I learned all of these things a little at a time while talking with the students.

Once I asked them, "Do your parents understand why you're here, leading this kind of life?"

"No," they answered. "We ignored their opposition and came anyway." Didn't they want to go back to the university so they could graduate?

"I'd like to go back," one of them said, "but since we're spending all this time here, I'll probably never graduate." Another said, "The university's not a place worth returning to." I admired their resolve, but I also remembered how much I had wanted to attend high school and wondered if they weren't wasting their opportunities.

Through these conversations, something within me gradually began to awaken. While these students had come to our village with no personal agenda, just to offer their support, I, who had sworn revenge against Chisso, hadn't yet taken a single significant step. I started to ask myself exactly what role I should play. It wasn't that the students told me to take any particular action. They didn't even invite me to join their movement. As outsiders, they acted prudently, so as not to alienate the villagers. They didn't do anything to call attention to themselves. They knew this was our fight and that they would have to stay in the background. Only when I told them about my personal hatred for Chisso and desire to destroy the company did they offer an opinion. There were many people who harbored the same feelings, they told me; rather than trying to fight alone, we should present a united front.

Before the students arrived there had already been a few activists among the patients. I was aware of these people, but at that time it was all I could do to heal the wounds I had created by leaving home, and to get used to my new lifestyle. Traditionally our region is known for its fierce political rivalries. Around election time, the sparks really fly. Even as a child I thought the whole thing was ridiculous. There was no real difference among the candidates; they all stood for the same thing. What was the point of voting when the only choices were a cunning badger and a sly fox? Probably the reason people here get so passionate during an election is that it's the only time their value to society is even minimally acknowledged. It's the only time you'll see a politician bow his head. It's the only time the villagers are treated as if they actually count. The candidates' support groups scramble to recruit villagers, while the villagers themselves become uneasy if they aren't affiliated with one camp or another.

Although I had become keenly interested in politics when I was an elementary school student, I knew even then that this type of local drama wasn't anything in which I wanted to participate. In my youthful idealism I sought a process born of greater sincerity and meaning. It was probably because I lived with the powerful influence of losing my father to such a dreadful disease that I believed that there must be a higher level of performance, a mechanism that dealt with real issues. With the death of my coastal fishing culture, I found myself caught up in a rising tide of social activism.

Social Activism

Before the decisive Kumamoto District Court ruling of 1973 decreeing that Chisso was responsible for compensation, the Minamata movement consisted of a variety of victims' groups, each with its own objectives. Though their goals might differ, however, there was a sense of unity among the groups in their fight against injustice and in their desire to expose all aspects of the Minamata tragedy to the general public. Up to this point, demands for compensation were secondary. But after the 1973 ruling, the focus of the movement shifted to certification of unrecognized patients. The administrative mechanism for certification was established, and eventually both victims and supporters were sucked into this system. In this way the whole movement gradually became institutionalized. The track was laid, so to speak, and we had to move on it.

In 1974 I presented my application for certification as a victim of Minamata disease to the governor of Kumamoto Prefecture, joined the Minamata Disease Certification Applicants' Council, and became deeply involved in their struggle. Fishing was put on hold. At my busiest, I would be away from home for half a month at a time doing work for the Applicants' Council. This was the beginning of a constant struggle with my extended family and other villagers over the fact that I wasn't living up to my responsibilities. Criticism from my family was painful. Although I felt I was doing the right thing, I could not provide any arguments in favor of this volunteer work, which didn't bring in a single yen.

Even the four students supporting the movement in my village seemed surprised to see me so involved. I would spend days debating and arguing with bureaucrats, policemen, and doctors. I soon became notorious for being confrontational and violent. I would arrive at government offices without an appointment and just walk in. If bureaucrats tried to avoid me, I would shower them with verbal abuse, kick them, or throw ashtrays.

In 1975 I was elected vice president of the Applicants' Council. At twenty-one, I felt somewhat inadequate for the position, but what was I to do? For the next six years I served as both vice president and secretary-general of the council. I would walk into the Prefectural Hall in Kumamoto City and present my demands. The staff of the Pollution Department was plagued by my presence, and it was rumored that its members prayed for the day when they would be transferred to another department. It was especially tough on lower-ranking officials, who tended to remain in one department for a long time. I can sympathize with them now.

I was careful not to meet with any of the officials alone, as I did not want to give the impression that I was conducting some under-the-table deal. I was also careful not to get cited for speeding or drunk driving. Even something like a traffic violation could be used against me, which would in turn hurt the council and the entire movement. However, I was always prepared to be arrested. I never compromised my political behavior for fear of arrest.

In 1975, a number of Minamata disease patients whose applications for certification had been rejected by Kumamoto Prefecture filed an appeal with the national Environment Agency in Tokyo. After reviewing their case, the Environment Agency overturned the prefecture's decision. This angered the prefecture, and a delegation was sent to Tokyo with a counterappeal. Prefectural representatives questioned why they should be obliged to recognize applicants that they did not consider victims. One member of the delegation, Assemblyman Sugimura Kunio, was quoted as saying, "Among the so-called Minamata disease patients there are quite a few fakes who are just trying to make some money."

After reading this statement in the newspaper, I got together with members of the Applicants' Council to discuss how we should respond to this outrageous remark. So it was that on September 25, 150 of us boarded three buses and drove to the Prefectural Assembly Hall. It was the day when the Special Committee on Pollution Countermeasures was conducting public hearings, and the committee chair happened to be Sugimura. Just at that time our council president and leader of the Minamata movement, Kawamoto Teruo, was visiting a group of Canadian Indians affected by mercury poisoning on a reservation near Kenora in Ontario. As a result, it fell to me to lead our protest.

When we arrived at the conference room, we found we had been preceded by fifty or more plainclothes policemen and five or six camera crews. The atmosphere was charged. Less than one hour after the meeting began a recess was called, and Sugimura and some others tried to rush out. I thought this was suspicious and asked someone to confirm that this was just a recess and that the meeting would continue. An official then had to admit that this was actually the end of the meeting. In other words, Sugimura and his companions had fled. We were right on their heels. Sugimura was in the hallway surrounded by guards, about to escape. We stopped them, and a big shoving match ensued between patients, officials, and guards.

To be honest, I didn't think that they would arrest me for this, but they did. The charges were assault and interference with a government official in the execution of his duties. It is true that I hit him, kicked him, and interfered with the execution of his duties, which at that time consisted of escaping. But it's equally true that they pulled some dirty tricks. Sugimura appeared on a news broadcast, sitting in a wheelchair with his head, legs, and arms so bandaged up that he looked like a mummy. I couldn't believe how much they had exaggerated his injuries. We found out that the prefectural police had set up a unit to investigate this incident the day before it happened. Another strange thing was that I was arrested more than ten days later. Normally, with this type of charge you would be arrested right on the spot. It was clear that the prefectural assembly and the police were trying to direct attention away from Sugimura's offensive statement about "fake victims of Minamata disease." Their objective was to depict our confrontation as violent, thereby damaging the reputation of our movement.

On the morning of October 7, I was shaken from my sleep as I lay in bed

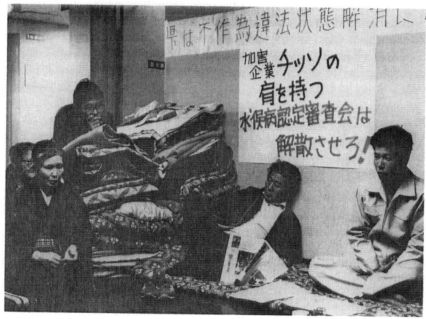

Masato (right) and Kawamoto (center) engage in a sit-in before the governor's office at Kumamoto Prefectural Hall (circa 1978).

on the second floor of the main house of the Ogata clan. I opened my eyes to many strange faces. I learned that fifty police officers had been dispatched to arrest me. Police cars had sped through wind and rain, prepared to surprise the village at the break of dawn. They circulated around the village, questioning residents about my activities. Apparently, this was designed to give the impression that I was a dangerous criminal. Three other people were arrested besides me. Handcuffed in the back of a police car, I began singing enka, in a loud, clear voice. Perhaps I was trying to bolster my courage with these popular songs, deeply rooted in regional traditions. Instead of scolding me, the police told me I was a good singer. "You don't know how lucky you are," I replied. "I usually perform only in big theaters, but today you can enjoy a free concert." It was during this period of arrest that I came to understand that the soul cannot be incarcerated. In my cell, I gazed at the guards. From their perspective, I was a captive. But in my mind, it was the guards who were trapped behind bars. Everything is relative.

I was detained by the police for seventeen days and then indicted, but I wasn't about to give up the fight. After all, it was we who were being poisoned and killed. My initial plan was to stand up in court and say, "Sure I did all those things—but why not? They deserved it!" My lawyers tried to dissuade me with the argument that while they understood how I felt, this approach was not going to go over in court. Nonetheless, I persisted. We had over forty hearings in the district court alone. Then the case was taken up to the Supreme Court. With each guilty verdict, my codefendants would start wavering. They couldn't bear to be seen as criminals by their own families and by society at large. "Look at the yakuza," I would encourage them. "They're proud of their criminal records. We should be proud that we got this verdict for fighting rather than running." Fifteen years passed before a final verdict was reached. I was judged guilty on two counts: preventing an official from carrying out his duties and inflicting injury upon a person. I received a suspended sentence. Now I am a man with a criminal record.

Our movement made its base camp at Soshisha, which means "Mutual Consideration Society." Soshisha is a small compound of buildings located on a hill in Minamata City, overlooking the Shiranui Sea. Soshisha was established in 1974 by Minamata disease patients and supporters with financial help from donors all over Japan. It was designed as a support facility for patients and their families, a place where they could discuss and work out their problems. The staff also worked to promote and coordinate social and scientific research on Minamata disease. Established in the wake of the first compensation agreement between certified patients and Chisso Company, Soshisha was concerned from the outset about problems likely to arise from this agreement. Organizers of Soshisha foresaw that after receiving compensation, the victims would lose the psychological support that they had had during the fight and become alienated from society. Soshisha offered a support system for the patients and a place where they could meet comfortably and help each other. This is how the place took on the name *soshi*, or caring for each other. One of our original goals was to create *moo hitotsu no sekai*, "another kind of world."

Members of our movement would spend the night at Soshisha several times a month, when our meetings lasted too late to return home, or when we were very tired, or when we'd been drinking far into the night. In fact the Applicants' Council came into existence soon after Soshisha was established.

This was a time when the focus of the whole Minamata movement shifted to the victims who were not yet certified, so it was easy for both Soshisha and the council to work together to address this common concern. Because both organizations were young, they were brimming with energy and hope. Most of the members were about my own age. Our strong sense of comradeship gave us the feeling that anything was possible. We weren't just fighting against Chisso but against the system itself; we were there to change the world. As we drank together we'd end up singing "The Internationale" and other labor songs. It was also a time of tension, with frequent confrontations

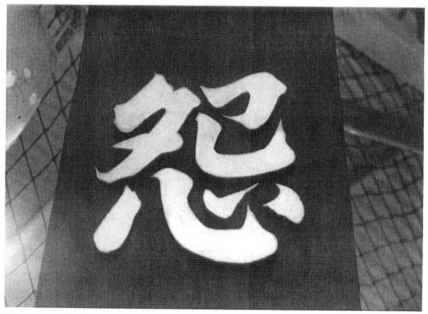

A banner used in the Minamata movement, with the character for urami, *signifying bitterness, grudge, and anger (Soshisha exhibit)*

with the police. We were summoned to appear in court, and the police came to our villages to question people about us. But I was firm in my convictions; I was determined to turn society around.

An important feature of the Minamata movement was that the victims' opinions always remained in the forefront, while the political views of their supporters remained hidden in the back. This was probably the result of a conscious effort by the older leaders, who had learned from experience. In other movements of the time, supporters and leftist political groups tended to dominate the cause, overshadowing the original message of those immediately affected. The elders in our group were especially careful not to fall into the pattern that had evolved in the movement against the construction of the New Tokyo International Airport in Narita. Following the government's decision in 1966 to construct a new airport in Chiba Prefecture, farmers in the village of Sanrizuka staged a large-scale protest movement against the appropriation of their land and homes. But farmers fighting to keep their land were overwhelmed by political groups with their own agendas. These outsiders ended up causing confusion and division among the protestors, weakening their struggle, which ultimately failed.

Another reason why outsiders remained marginal in the Minamata movement was that left-wing activists, with their Marxist class-struggle orientation, found it hard to adapt their ideological framework to industrial pollution and the rights of its victims. Moreover, underlying the Minamata disease incident was a long and intricate history of social relations and rich local traditions. Unless the supporters had the patience and diligence to study this social history, there was no way they could become a part of regional society or manipulate the Minamata disease issue for their own ideological purposes.

Throughout Japan there was an expression, "Minamata in the West and Narita in the East." As this expression tells us, Minamata had become a networking center for activists concerned with human rights, environmental protection, and industrial responsibility. Activists came to visit from all over Japan. Our movement established ties with citizens' movements concerned with a variety of issues related to irresponsible development and environmental destruction. These included the construction of a new thermal-electric power plant in Oita, the construction of a crude-oil storage facility in Kagoshima, land reclamation in Nagasaki, the Kanemi cooking oil PCB poisoning incident, and so on.[2] We were also in close touch with the Buraku Liberation League, which fights discrimination against this "outcaste" group of some three million people. Our growing understanding of their situation shed light on the human-rights aspect of our own fight.[3]

*   *   *

As you can see, I became deeply involved in the Minamata movement, but had it not been for the inspiration of the late Kawamoto Teruo, I probably would not have committed myself so wholeheartedly. Kawamoto had been leading the movement for a number of years before I became active. He was born on August 1, 1932, placing him a generation ahead of me. After I joined the movement, we were the two central figures. We hit it off really well and had some fine times together. I was impressed that even in our region there was a man who was not afraid to confront government officials or the company. He was willing to bare his soul before the authorities without fear of arrest, giving me the courage to do the same. Here was someone I could follow and learn from, I thought. Especially during the first few years, people often commented on the nice dynamic between us. Of course we took other people's opinions into consideration, but it was our discussions that constituted the core of the movement.

Kawamoto told me that in his younger days he worked in the coal mines and also as a day laborer. Around 1971, he worked as a nurse. He had gone to nursing school and had become licensed. In those days male nurses were still pretty unusual. His father, a fisherman, had died of Minamata disease, and Kawamoto himself was a certified patient. He became famous in the early history of Minamata disease for tracking down new victims and encouraging patients to step forward and receive assistance. He negotiated on their behalf with government agencies and with Chisso Company. I'm pretty forward by nature. I've never feared or deferred to anyone just because they were older than I am. Kawamoto and I were both radical, but I was definitely the more confrontational.

As I became embroiled in court cases, it wasn't unusual for me to make as many as two trips per month to Tokyo. At first everything seemed confusing, but I gradually grasped the jargon and the procedure. I've never learned things through books; instead I rely on direct experience. When I didn't understand a word I would look it up in the dictionary or ask someone. I knew it would weaken our case if I used the wrong words in public statements, so I went out of my way to expand my vocabulary. What you learn through necessity sticks with you. This is true not only about language but of legal and political tactics. Just before a hearing or a trial we would stay up late and plan our strategy. I became pretty knowledgeable about our opponents' tactics. The bureaucrats knew how to talk without saying anything meaningful and how to dominate the floor so that we couldn't find an opening to express our views. I thoroughly enjoyed those moments when I succeeded in staging surprise attacks and creating openings in which we ourselves might speak. Sometimes we were so effective that the opposition ended up looking like victims. I was developing into quite a strategist.

In 1981 I was elected president of the Applicants' Council. It was our

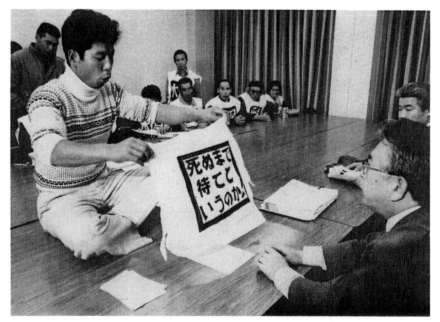

Masato confronts government officials at Kumamoto Prefectural Hall, with a banner that reads, "Are you telling us to wait until we die?" (circa 1983)

group that first took the national government to court, demanding that the state itself acknowledge responsibility for the Minamata incident. One of the key points pursued by our group was the government's deliberate delay in certifying patients with Minamata disease. Especially after 1980, our group focused on a court case regarding administrative negligence on the part of the prefectural governor. In social welfare cases, decisions must be handed down within three months of the application date. In the case of Minamata disease certification, however, the prefecture was not bound by any time limit for its response. Applicants had to wait for an inordinately long time. In the mid-1970s the court had agreed that the process should be expedited, but because a definite time limit was not established, the ruling had no binding power. Having no other recourse, we demanded that so many cases be handled per year. However, this didn't mean that the applicant would be certified. By the 1980s the number of successful applicants had dropped significantly. While in the 1970s about 70 percent of applicants were being certified, only about 10 percent were certified in the early 1980s. It was obvious that the government was manipulating criteria for its own purposes. Under my leadership we initiated a court battle against the state, demanding a new process that would replace the old certification policies.

Life Changes

I was married in May of 1977. Before I said my vows, I told my bride, "I want you to know that my first wife is the Minamata movement. . . . And no matter what anyone says, even if the sun should rise from the west, the movement has first priority," I added. My wife was a schoolmate from junior high. Since we knew each other pretty well, I didn't really think we needed to go through the traditional formality of having a *nakodo*, or go-between, who negotiates between the two families. But when I learned that her parents had found someone to represent them, I had to ask my uncle to represent me. Her parents had their *nakodo* approach my uncle with a condition for our marriage: I had to quit the movement. My uncle felt obliged to come over and try to persuade me, but he knew how stubborn I was. "Listen, Masato," he said. "Traditionally a *nakodo* is forgiven a few lies in order to get a couple together. Let's just pretend that I heard you say you planned to quit the movement. They can't really blame me later if they find out it was a lie. All we need here is a little white lie." "Well, if you think it's all right to lie, it's your responsibility," I replied. I knew the lie wouldn't hold up for three days. Later I told the other *nakodo*, "There isn't one person in this world who can change my mind. My own family certainly hasn't been successful—so you might as well forget it."

I was born stubborn, and I'll probably never change. I was so deeply involved in the movement that I couldn't imagine quitting. I thought that if I quit I would lose my identity—I would no longer be myself. It's like having a sake bottle sitting in front of you, and people tell you to pretend it doesn't exist. Once I had seen it, how could I pretend it didn't exist? My family often said, "Why does it have to be you who's so involved in all these things?" But if I didn't do them, who would? "Is there something wrong with what I'm doing?" I asked them. But no one was willing to say I was actually wrong or mistaken in my actions, so I pressed on. I always tried to break down opposition by confronting people directly.

Eventually the villagers stopped criticizing me. But that didn't mean they understood what I was doing. They just decided that what I was doing was useless and became indifferent. Had I been making money, I would have had their full support, but I was giving myself to the movement precisely because my efforts were rewarded by something other than money. In the eighties the entire world seemed to be obsessed with money. I was going against the flow. Although I was leading a group that fought for financial compensation, on a personal level I found money increasingly meaningless. This contradiction would take its toll.

I thought I would never be interested in fame and social status. But after serving as vice president, and then president, of the Applicants' Council, I felt a certain pride and sense of responsibility. I can't deny that it felt good to be in a position of leadership. This unexpected manifestation of ego troubled me.

Physically, too, I was not in the best of shape. Throughout the years I dedicated to the movement, I had had many health problems related to Minamata disease. I had a terrible time with numbness in my arms and hands, legs and feet, and in my head. Often my legs and arms would shake uncontrollably, and there was a constant ringing in my ears. Especially when I would lie down to sleep, my entire body, from my feet to my shoulders, would stiffen with cramps, throwing the people around me into a panic.

As I look back on it now, I can see that from the early 1980s the atmosphere at Soshisha began to change. In fact, this seems to have been a time when the approaches taken by citizens' movements nationwide began to evolve. First of all, activists—including myself—were getting older and had family responsibilities. Moreover, the movement had shifted from the streets to the courts. We now found ourselves occupied with bureaucratic procedures and paperwork. We were locked into the system. Soshisha itself was undergoing a financial crisis. In its early years it had been run on donations, but the time had come for it to be financially independent. In order to finance their cause, Soshisha's activists had to become businessmen. We began to produce and distribute mushrooms and *amanatsu,* sweet summer *mikan.* As a member of the Fruit Growers Association of Minamata Patient Families, I produced over four tons of *mikan* for Soshisha.

In 1983 and 1984 I worked as a salesman for a propane gas company in the town of Sashiki. It had become impossible to make a living by fishing. I had tried fish-farming with red snapper, but the business wasn't sufficient to make ends meet, so we often depended on help from my mother. As a certified Minamata disease patient, my mother had been receiving compensation money. Because our life was pretty miserable, and my pride wouldn't allow me to keep accepting help from my mother—especially when it came from compensation funds—I decided to get an outside job. For many years I had been feeling guilty that I had neglected my family in favor of the movement. In this sense, returning to the life of an employee may have been a form of penance. I also sought to regain some of the discipline I had learned in the past from working under other people.

At the outset, I decided that I would seek employment for no more than two years. I was still involved in the movement, and at first journalists would even stop by the office. My boss told me that this couldn't go on, because it interfered with our work. This was the only incident that took place between me and the company in the two some years I worked there. I was a pretty hard worker, if I say so myself. I was a good salesman, too. I brought in a lot of new customers to buy our propane products. Although I was also very busy with work related to the compensation movement, I only took off two or three days per month. I always made up the time by filling in on my holidays, when other workers were absent.

Every day I arrived at work earlier than everyone. Whenever I embark on something new, I make a promise to myself. This time, it was never to be late to work. I arrived, at the latest, fifteen minutes before the shop opened. Sometimes I would be there two or three hours before the office opened. The manager was amazed. The other employees didn't seem to have any qualms about arriving late. They always had one excuse or another—the kids were sick, there was a traffic jam, and so on. The boss never got angry with them. I think he was afraid that if he made too many demands, his employees would quit, and he knew how hard they would be to replace. It was a tough job for the money he was paying. After all, we had to lug heavy propane canisters along mountain trails too narrow for our truck. Usually I ignored the other workers, but sometimes their bad attitudes really got to me, and I would tell them off. They had no idea what I was talking about. As long as they were receiving a salary, nothing else mattered. This might have been the modern work ethic, but I just couldn't get used to it. Sometimes I would even shout at the manager's son, who was being groomed to take over the business. I was governed by two principles: I should work as hard as I could, but it didn't matter when I quit. I wasn't afraid of being fired for expressing my beliefs.

During my two years at the company I was late only once. A customer called complaining that his water heater wasn't working well. So I told him I'd be there first thing in the morning to fix it. I had gone without telling my boss, and naturally I was late to work. When I arrived at work I felt a strange tension—someone was late who had never been late before. Still, I didn't explain myself to anyone. Apparently one of the women clerks who had heard the phone call come in a few days before explained the situation to the manager. "Why didn't you just tell me?" he asked. I replied that the fact that I didn't offer an excuse should show that I had a legitimate reason. My boss was dumbfounded by this response, and I was shocked that he couldn't grasp such simple logic. I found myself in a similar situation a few years later when I quit the movement. I made no excuses and gave no explanations. People who know me well always tell me I make my life more difficult because of this trait.

After two years I resigned from the company, as I had planned. The owner tried to persuade me to stay and offered to give me a raise. Although I was grateful to him, I couldn't accept. I had set my goals, and I wouldn't break them. I was happy to leave the company without any bad feelings. The manager and I are still good friends today. His son is now the owner, and he tells me that he understands why I was so hard on him. "Those were good lessons," he admits.

Leaving the Movement

All of the turning points in my life have appeared to me as well-lit crossroads. Facing my father's death, running away from home, deciding to return, becoming involved in the Minamata movement, leaving the movement— each juncture was marked by deep thought and anguish, as I sought to define my position and take the right course. But once I made up my mind, I never had any regrets. It gives me confidence to know that I have always been true to my beliefs and have never had any need to flee my own conscience. Were this not the case, my life would be worthless.

In 1985, two years after I left the propane job, I had to face the fact that I now had three children to support and that my life was a shambles. It was all because of the movement. "Isn't a man in his twenties and thirties supposed to be at the height of his working life, supporting a family?" my wife and mother would complain. My mother was especially persistent. When I came out of the bathroom, she would be standing at the door, ready to attack. As I sat down at a meal, she would sit next to me and lecture me about my life. It was always the same thing, day after day, year after year. My wife and I quarreled all the time. Sometimes I would listen quietly, but at other times I would blow up. I thought that one day they would finally understand, and I kept telling myself that if I were just patient long enough, things would work out. But as I look back on those days, I realize that it was precisely because I had such strong resistance from my family that I reached the point that I could question my involvement with the Minamata disease movement. If my mother and wife had encouraged my participation, I wouldn't have held out so long, and I probably wouldn't have reached the level of spiritual growth I have attained today.

My mother used to say to me, "Everything will be fine if you just catch fish, grow sweet potatoes and greens, and eat your fill." She was trying to tell me that I should be content with the kind of life my family had always led. However hard I might work in the movement, it would not put food on the table

91

and would most definitely not bring my father back. My mother didn't speak from some solid philosophical foundation. These were simply words distilled from her everyday life in the small world she had lived in since the day she was born. When she first uttered this advice it depressed me that she was such a narrow-minded country hick, with no knowledge of the outside world.

Later, after I experienced a period of mental agony and revelation, these words came back to me with new meaning and relevance. Stop running around looking for life, she was saying. It's right here at home. Let national politics take their course. The answer isn't in Tokyo but here. This is where you belong, said those words—right here, facing the ocean and the mountains.

It wasn't just my family who criticized me but the entire village. Although my neighbors didn't speak out directly, as we had lived in the same village all of our lives, I knew exactly how they felt. For example, the day after my name had been mentioned on television or appeared in the newspaper, I could see the same question in their eyes, "What's the point?" For these people the only meaningful element of the Minamata movement was monetary compensation. There was nothing beyond it. They could understand my involvement within this framework. They couldn't understand that someone might be involved in the movement on behalf of people other than themselves.

If I were to abandon the movement and let it deteriorate, how could I face my father in the next life? But it became ever more clear that once the victims were certified and received compensation they would cease fighting, and that once they had stepped into the background, our story would be erased from the public mind. Did this mean that in the last analysis, the Minamata disease victims could be purchased and silenced with yen, that the movement itself was about nothing more than money? It seemed that no one wanted to address the more important issues. But the problem was that not even I could clearly identify those issues.

I began to have doubts. If I wasn't in the movement for money, was I in it to avenge my father's death? What would happen after I had realized that revenge? Was it just an illusion to entertain the thought that I was putting the interest of others above my own? How could I pretend to be altruistic when I was making my own family suffer? Did the end justify the means? Bombarded by these questions, I could no longer function normally.

As we approached the thirtieth anniversary of the "discovery" of Minamata disease, the movement was foundering. It no longer had direction. Activists were caught up in day-to-day problems. With each court case we fought, we thought we were making progress, but it was this very sense of progress that blinded us. We were too busy to realize that we no longer had a master plan to guide us into the future. One of the most frustrating aspects of dealing with the government, whether at the local, prefectural, or national level, was that the people in charge constantly changed, and we had to cover the same ground over and over again. There seemed to be no end in sight. We would have to sue the compensation board for being too slow in granting compensation. For that we would seek compensation. So it became compensation on top of compensation. Whatever we did, wherever we went, whomever we dealt with, the only common language was money, and unless we could translate everything into this language, it was as if we could no longer communicate. It was like trying to run through mud that was getting deeper and deeper.

By then my relationship with Kawamoto Teruo had become strained. I felt that Kawamoto was interested in dealing with the Minamata issue only within the framework of the government system. He continued to be resourceful as we developed new strategies for court cases, appeals, filings, motions, and other political and legal measures. We were in the center of a whirlpool of activity, but it was as if we no longer remembered whom we were fighting. There was no attempt to face Chisso head-on. When I suggested that we reassess our tactics and face Chisso directly, Kawamoto disagreed, on the grounds that this would invite political isolation. During this time Kawamoto ran for the city council and won a seat on his second attempt. It seemed to me that he was growing increasingly conservative and was reluctant to engage in direct confrontation.

We spent so much time in court that the legal system was wearing me down. No matter who won a case, there were always appeals. What was more important, we found ourselves becoming part of the system and bureaucracy that we had set out to fight. We could not fight the system unless we were in it. Our court briefs and political statements were full of technical words and political jargon. Although our movement had grown in size, most of the work was done by a small core. In court cases our general members were needed only as faceless numbers. The only time we called upon them was to place their seals on court documents. Lawyers and movement leaders saved the general membership from experiencing the battlefield. We led the membership in whatever direction we pleased. We had come to resemble our government counterparts.

In those days Kawamoto's opinion still held sway, and next to him I must have looked pretty radical. Our conflict was beginning to have a negative effect on the membership. Sooner or later the members would be forced to choose between us. I had seen many other movements fail because of internal conflicts among the leadership. On the other hand, I couldn't compromise my own views. So, in September, when my term as president of the Applicants' Council was about to expire, I decided to leave the movement.

The Depths of Despair

After submitting my resignation to the Applicants' Council, I spent three days wandering along the reedy shore of Sashiki River. I waded through the water and sat on a sand spit for hours, thinking and sobbing in agony. I felt that I had lost everything. I no longer knew who I was. I was assailed by questions I couldn't answer.

In the midst of this confusion, however, I realized that I couldn't just run away. I needed to make a clean break. I owed an explanation and word of thanks to those who had stood by me in the movement. I felt especially bad about the way I had left things with Kawamoto. I wanted to thank him for all he had done for me, to tell him I had no hard feelings. But it wasn't that easy. We were no longer on speaking terms. Still, I told myself, if I didn't try, I would always regret it.

After agonizing about this for some time, I decided to ask Yanagida Koichi, a friend from Soshisha, to accompany me to Kawamoto's place. During my years in the movement lots of people frequented my house, but it must have been Yanagida who came over most often. He had come to Minamata as a supporter and ended up settling there. "I understand how you feel," he said, "but I don't think I'm prepared to leave with you." "That's fine," I replied. I was just happy that he had answered me so directly and honestly. He was the only person who told me how he really felt.

That's why, when I was worrying about how to approach Kawamoto, I thought that Yanagida might be able to help. He agreed, but he said he doubted that Kawamoto would understand my feelings. I can remember very clearly what I said then. "I don't know whether I'll be able to make myself understood, either, but I have to try. Even among carpenters and plasterers, when an apprentice is ready to go off on his own, there is a proper way to bid farewell."

For me, this truly was the end of an apprenticeship. I had learned so much from Kawamoto. He had been so generous in guiding me. The gulf between us would probably remain, and we would probably go our separate ways, but it was my duty to meet with him again.

It was a short visit. Kawamoto was filing newspaper clippings and wouldn't even look up at me. The only thing I managed to say was, "Kawamoto-*san*, I don't think we'll find any gods or buddhas in the afterworld. Don't you think they are all living with us right here in this life?" Kawamoto looked incredulous. He didn't seem to grasp a word. But I felt there was nothing I could add.

I think that what I was trying to say to him is that our chance for reunion exists only in this world. I wanted to heal our relationship while we both lived. I don't blame him for not understanding me. I was losing touch with reality. My words were no longer logical.

Although I was telling Kawamoto that we could find a solution only in this life, I was already teetering dangerously between this world and the next. Death became a temptation. Was it true that solutions could be found only now while we live? Or, could we find salvation only after death? In this world, or the other? While we live, or after we die? I was battered by self-doubt.

I never held any bitter feelings toward Kawamoto. If I had felt anger or bitterness, I probably would not have lost my mind. If I had hated Kawamoto or others in the movement, they would have become the target of my emotions. Instead, I turned upon myself. Everything was focused within, on the questions I couldn't even ask, on the search for something I couldn't even identify. I had nothing to lean on; I couldn't see ahead. I went crazy.

After I visited Kawamoto, I traveled to Tokyo, Nagoya, Osaka, and Kyoto to offer my thanks and bid goodbye to friends and supporters in the Applicants' Council. This was part of the process of breaking away. By the end of the trip it was obvious that I was suffering a nervous breakdown. I barely made it home.

All of this took place in September 1985. By this time I was also ready to withdraw my application for certification as a Minamata disease patient. I had long been saying that I wasn't fighting for money. "Then, for what?" people had asked. Now I was asking myself the same question. But I just couldn't seem to find the answer.

From the time I decided to withdraw my application until December, when I actually went through the process of withdrawal, I went mad. While I was debating what I should do, I was suffering, but I still had control of my mind. Usually when you let go of one support system or goal, you have another in view. I saw a blank wall.

You ask, what was the most painful aspect of this period? I'd have to say it was the loneliness. No one understood my position—not Kawamoto, with whom I had once shared so much, or my other friends, or my mother, or my wife. I had never felt so alone in my whole life. Up to a point, I could have changed my mind. With a simple apology to council members I could have returned to my old life. But somehow I had enough strength to keep plodding along.

Those three months seemed like thirty years. It was a long road. There were so many times I thought that this was it, there was no point in living any longer. But just when I was on the brink, something new and strange would happen.

When does a nervous breakdown begin? At what point do you lose your mind? It's not that clear. It seemed to begin right about the time I was talking on the phone with Tsuchimoto Noriaki, known for his excellent documentaries on Minamata disease. I was providing him with names of people deeply involved in the Minamata movement, when I started babbling about the meaning of their names. "Kawamoto means that rivers, *kawa*, are the basis, *moto*, for everything. Your name means that soil, *tsuchi*, is the origin of all things. My friend Yanagida Koichi's name means that he cultivates rice fields. Ishimure Michiko's name has the character *michi*, suggesting that she walks the path of humanity." My point was that people's names reveal the way they live, their hopes and prayers. I realized how simplistic I was being, but I wanted to get at something more fundamental than philosophy and ideology. "Yes, yes, quite right," agreed Tsuchimoto kindly. My own name always embarrasses me: "Masato" means "righteous person." Adults were always telling me to live up to my name. When my mother scolded me, I used to tell her, "It's all your fault for giving me this terrible name. Why didn't you just call me 'the bad one'?"

One of my earliest symptoms was insomnia. Even at night my head remained clear, and I couldn't sleep. I remember thinking that this was odd. I seemed to be on a high all day. I was hyperactive. My internal clock seemed to shut down. Even when I was physically exhausted, my mind was still alert. Sometimes I would suddenly fall into a deep sleep and awaken feeling that I must have slept for hours. Then my watch would tell me it had only been five minutes. When I felt that I really should get some sleep, I would drink a whole bottle of *shochu*. Even then, I couldn't fall asleep. In this condition, it was impossible to work.

Soon everything I tried to do became a big ordeal. I couldn't even eat a bowl of rice without crying. I would wonder, how many living things were in that bowl? How many of them was I eating? If I could have talked about my feelings, I would have felt much better, but the words wouldn't come. Eventually I couldn't eat at all. Fish is my favorite food, but I couldn't eat it. For a long time I ate only rice gruel and *umeboshi*, green plums pickled in salt. I didn't have any consciousness of eating; it was as if I were feeding someone else.

I spent a lot of time walking the beaches and river banks, or wandering through the hills and fields. I also paid many visits to my father's grave, up on a bluff behind our house. I had no consciousness of losing my mind; I was simply intent on thinking, on searching. I was obsessed with a question: Why, in the last analysis, do people always fall for money? If not money, what? I also tried to make sense of our social system and the emperor system. I was always lost in thought, but regardless of the topic, one phrase kept surfacing like a refrain: If not money, what? My family tried to put me in a mental institution. "This all comes from your obsession with Minamata disease," grumbled my mother.

What concerned me the most were connections—links that would connect me to the world. Having cut all normal ties, it would be up to me to establish new ones. Because I was so concerned about relationships, I can remember exactly what my family went through, what they said to me, and how I answered. When my wife and children saw me in anguish, they suffered the same pain. Knowing how much suffering I was causing them made things even more difficult for me.

It was early October, sometime before the nights turn cool. It must have been about 11:30 P.M. Suddenly I was overcome with revulsion for my television. I grabbed the TV, pushed my wife aside, and went out the door, muttering something like, "I've got to get rid of this." I hurled the television into the front garden and screamed, "You beast! How dare you break into my house and order us around. Go there! Buy this! Dress like that! Telling all kinds of lies, spewing out all kinds of bullshit! I know who you are!" I grabbed one of the decorative rocks in the garden and smashed the screen. "Now look at you," I said with satisfaction, thinking that with this I could draw my family back to me.

It didn't stop with the television. I couldn't tolerate being surrounded by machines. I would deliberately run the car off onto rocky hillsides, smashing up the body. After my wife had it repaired at a body shop, I would go out and smash it up some more. People asked me why I was wasting so much money, but I was desperate. It was as if I had awakened one day to find that machines were pressing in on us from all sides. I needed to draw a clear line between people and these mechanical objects. Either I would destroy them, or they would destroy me. I felt that I was regaining my sanity; others thought my mind was slipping more all the time.

Facing My Demons

One day it dawned on me that I was being tested. It was like passing the halfway point on a mountain climb. To get this far, you trudge along, eyes to the ground, oblivious to everything around you. Then suddenly you can see the view. I was beginning to see that everything is interrelated. I hadn't taken this path of my own volition. I was being directed along this course. Nothing in my life had been meaningless. Everything I had done had led me to this point. This was no ordinary illness, I decided.

Pieces of the past fit into place, but I was still uncertain about the future. There were so many times that I had come through, only to discover that I was still in doubt, still assailed by endless questions. But answers to these questions also began to take shape. Grass, trees, birds, sea, fish, human gestures and words—expressions of nature to which I had grown indifferent—all seemed to offer subtle hints. Then, before I knew it, one set of hints would open up into another, as if I was turning the lens of a kaleidoscope. Even shapes, colors, and sounds offered hints.

I was drawn to the hills. When I spoke to the trees, they would answer. Of course, they didn't use human words. It was more like the voice of the wind, explaining to me in one more way what it meant to be alive. I was participating in a communion of living spirits, in an exchange of feelings unencumbered by words. Once, when I was walking near my father's grave, I heard the sound of water deep in the ground. This happened on a day when someone happened to be drilling for water in my neighborhood. I asked him to drill in the area where I had heard the water. My family was pretty skeptical. Most of the water in our area has a very high salt content, and dozens of people have tried to drill for water, all unsuccessfully. I was so confident, though, that the drilling team decided to take my advice. After drilling for fifty meters, they went through a rock formation and encountered an underground stream. It was wonderful water. I don't know exactly how I heard the water. It was a kind of organic communication.

I began to put things into perspective. I realized that even money, of which

I had spoken so negatively, had evolved with human beings. At first it may have taken the form of shells or stones; later we began to use iron and copper. Today it plays an integral role in human society. The world was a web of inevitability, of which I was a part. I was stunned to realize that I was related to everything.

The most important lesson, perhaps, was learning that interconnection included links to the past, to the deceased. In modern society we no longer feel any connection with the dead. But in fact, our souls are always connected. During my nervous breakdown I was always conscious of their presence—not as tangible beings but as a spiritual essence, alive in my heart. This is hard to explain, but I am sure that there must be many other people who have had similar experiences.

I was terrified. Processing all of these hints was draining; I was reaching the limits of concentration. But what if the messages should stop coming? What would I do then? I was exhausted and afraid. I no longer had any control over myself. I couldn't speak. I couldn't foresee what would happen in the next few seconds. I was trapped in a world beyond my control. I couldn't achieve anything through my own will—not even such basic functions as urinating, defecating, or sleeping. The only time I felt free from fatigue was in those few moments after awakening from a long sleep. Then my surroundings would launch another assault on my mind, pounding me with endless stimuli. Would I be able to survive another experience like this? I doubted it.

You know the expression, "Under a layer of skin is a different person." In my case, it was really true. Sometimes my skin would tingle, and my muscles would ripple uncontrollably. I've experienced spasms and convulsions, but this was much worse. I've been told that my eyes had an orange glow. I thought that my time had come. My wife tells me that I grasped her hand and traced the character *hito* (person) onto her palm. I remember this only faintly. "Do you mean that you want me to live like a human being?" my wife had asked. She said that I nodded in reply.

It was soon after that incident that I saw "Devil's Island." You know, it's the place the Peach Boy goes to recover stolen treasure in the folktale *Momotaro*. I wouldn't call it a dream or an illusion. It was invisible to other people, but I could see it. Not unlike the Peach Boy, who decides to go to the island to conquer devils, I was going to Chisso to face my demons. I saw myself descending by rope into a well-like structure until I found a horizontal passageway. At the end of the tunnel were four or five demons devouring something with relish. It was a human being. They were tearing off its limbs, and blood ran from their mouths as they chewed. Next to them was a pile of human remains.

Horrified, I began screaming. They were after me. By the time I reached the vertical shaft, the demons were right on my heels. At the last second my voice returned, and I screamed, "I'm a human being!" With that, a bright light shot out of me and blinded the demons, giving me a chance to escape up the shaft. At the top my father and other deceased villagers were waiting around the hole to pull me out. Some were uttering words of relief, and some were lecturing me. "That was close!" "We warned you about going to that place." I heard one of them ask, "Whose son is that?" "He's Fukumatsu's boy," another answered.

Around this time, there was another strange incident. I became obsessed with the image that Chisso was again dumping toxic waste into the ocean. One morning, while it was still dark, I dashed out of the house. I don't know how I managed to drive in that state of mind, not to mention the fact that I had been forbidden to drive at all. I hurried to the home of Tani Yoichi, one of the movement supporters and a friend of mine, who lived in the nearby village of Akasaki. Barging into his house, I told Tani that there was an emergency and we had to stop Chisso. Then I ran back out and began filling my car with stones. From Tani's viewpoint, I was nuts. He tried to hold me still and calm me, but to no avail.

Finally he said, "OK, I'll go with you." But he insisted on driving his own car. I thought we were going straight to Chisso, but he drove right by the turn off and headed for Soshisha. "Let's get those guys to join us," he said. We arrived just as dawn was breaking and startled everyone awake. I heard later that while they were trying to pacify me, they called a doctor they knew to ask his advice.

I finally gave in and said I'd do whatever they wanted. Next Yanagida took the wheel. Without telling me our destination, he drove me to a hospital in Hitoyoshi. As we drove, I gazed at the sunrise through the window. I felt that this was my last view of the world. Yanagida tried to make me feel better by talking about all sorts of different things. I appreciated his compassion, but I also didn't want to show any signs of weakness. By the time we entered Ama-zuki Tunnel, I had calmed down. I imagined that Kuma River, at the mouth of the tunnel, must be the River Styx. I was determined to go quietly. Some time after we had passed the river, I realized that I was starving. I guess this was proof that I still wished to live. We stopped at a drive-in restaurant, and although it wasn't open yet, Yanagida begged them to give us some food. All they could offer was miso soup and rice, but to me it was a feast.

I don't know how many days I stayed in the hospital. I just remember how badly I wanted to go home. Sometimes I accused Yanagida and my wife of wanting to imprison me. Thinking about it later, I realized that great num-bers of people have been placed in mental institutions against their will. But, what frightens me most is the kind of person that can live in this world without ever going crazy.

Eventually even I realized that I had crossed the peak of my illness. I felt an incredible sense of liberation. But this elation lasted no more than four or five days. I soon realized that having reached the top of the mountain, I would have to climb down the other side. The descent would be easier, but my trials were not yet over. I was still being assailed by all kinds of stimuli, but I felt that they were teaching me many things.

Gradually I regained my appetite and my ability to speak with people. It must have been in the second half of November that I felt an incredible urge to return to fishing, to return to the sea. It wasn't that I considered fishing a job. I simply wanted to go out and talk to the fish and the crabs, to see them again, like old friends. Just as my family experienced my suffering, they also felt the return of my health. My recovery progressed smoothly.

One day in December, I awakened from a nap in the back bedroom. My eyes opened and at that moment—I'll never forget this—a strange haiku-like poem entered my head.

> Awakened from a short nap,
> I return to reality.

With that, I was pushed back into the world. My body felt light. Normally I would have been overcome almost instantly by outside stimuli, but this time a minute passed, then three, then five. I can't describe how relieved and happy I felt. At the same time, I was amazed at how much was revealed to me during that seemingly interminable period of illness. I wanted to share my experiences with others, but I had no idea where to begin. On the one hand I felt relieved, while on the other I was afraid. What if the whole process started up again? Once taken captive, escape couldn't possibly be so simple. And there was always the lingering question—why did this happen to *me?*

There is one point I want to make clear. Some people interpreted my experience as a form of enlightenment, but I didn't see it that way. I knew that life would continue to have its ups and downs. A steady state would bore me. I want to keep searching, to keep riding the swells. I will never cease to be fascinated by what I went through. It was as if I had entered a spiritual dimension. I prefer to interpret it as a period of madness. The character for "madness" is written with the graph for "beast" on the left side and the graph for "king" on the right. I was truly both a beast and a king.

Tokoyo no fune, Boat to the Eternal World

On December 27, I went to Kumamoto City to withdraw my application for certification as a Minamata disease victim. There was a reason why I waited for more than three months after quitting the movement to do this. Early on I had explained my intentions to movement activists, but they pressed me to wait until a court verdict was issued on the alleged negligence of the state to act in a swift and timely manner in certifying the applicants. We had been asking for compensation for this delay, and because I had been representing the plaintiffs, it would not look good if I withdrew my application before the decision was made. I didn't want to put myself above the welfare of the group. The court's decision was favorable, but our request for forty thousand yen per month was reduced to twenty thousand yen. Later this was reduced even farther in the Court of Appeals.

I explained my decision to withdraw my application to my wife, but I'm not sure how well she understood me. She didn't say a word. She knew me too well to believe that anyone's opinion would change my mind. Even though I was contributing no more to the family than before, once I left the movement my mother finally stopped bombarding me with complaints and criticisms. But when I went off to withdraw my application, she couldn't help saying, "What a waste." She wasn't alone. People who had complained about my involvement in the movement were now telling me that if I had not withdrawn my application I at least could have made some money.

At the Prefectural Hall the atmosphere was "business as usual." I had called in advance, saying, "I'd like to discuss a personal matter of great importance, so I would appreciate some of your time." There were three or four officials there to meet with me. I handed them a letter explaining why I had decided to withdraw my application. In essence, I wrote that I had given up on them, that I had realized that the only person who could recognize my condition was myself. After that, I spoke with them for one or two hours. Now that I had withdrawn, we all felt at ease and were able to talk about a number of things. Then I asked them whether, just personally and

103

off the record, they believed that I was a victim of Minamata disease. "Yes," they said. We all laughed.

That was a moment of great satisfaction for me. I felt I had gone beyond them. My withdrawal should have pleased them, but they didn't look victorious. Instead, they wore an expression I hadn't seen before. They seemed to have reached their limits. It wasn't simply that they were confused as officials; they were confronting something new as individuals. I had always faced them as officials, wearing their formal masks of politeness and uttering their official lines. This time my words had penetrated the masks, revealing human faces. I was no longer a member of the movement but Ogata Masato; they were no longer officials but individual human beings. I still run into them from time to time, and I am always conscious of a special understanding between us.

As I welcomed the New Year of 1986, I became increasingly confident that I was in control of my mental faculties. However, the process of recovery was much more gradual than I thought it would be.

To mark the New Year, I wrote an open letter to Chisso and delivered it by hand as soon as everyone returned to work. It wasn't that I expected my letter to solve any problems. It simply represented a new direction for me; I wanted to confront Chisso on a direct and personal level. Chisso responded, but I told them their response was inadequate. Then, to give greater expression to my own feelings, I decided to build a wooden boat. I would sail this boat to Chisso, and there I would bear witness to what they had done. It would take time, though, to develop my plans. To begin with, it was almost impossible to find a place that would build a wooden boat. It took me a year to locate a boat builder and place an order. It took another six months to build the boat, and yet another half year before I could set sail.

How did I come up with this idea? I pictured the Minamata River flowing by the Chisso plant, and the effluent running into the river from the factory canal. Then I imagined myself rowing up river toward the source of the effluent, as if to push it back. If Chisso was the source of death, then the Shiranui Sea was the source of life. That was the main reason I wanted to go. I also wanted to reconfirm to myself that I would always be there, face to face with Chisso. Chisso was both my starting point and the stage where I would carry out my life struggle. I realized that I would always be a part of Chisso and a part of the system from which I tried to divorce myself.

Why did I insist that the boat be made of wood? It was because I would find it repugnant to go in a car or boat made from reinforced plastic. After all, such plastics had formed the mainstay of Chisso's income. Once made, plastics cannot return to the earth. If you go fishing, you'll see what I mean. Plastic garbage covers the sea. Until about thirty years ago, wooden boats were common in this region. I wanted to impart the message that it might be good to measure the present against my father's days.

Tokoyo, "the Eternal World." It's a fine name, don't you think? It does embarrass me just a little, since I'm a simple country fellow. But it's the name I picked out when I ordered the boat. The place I reached during my period of madness—that was the Eternal World. *Tokoyo* is a state of mind, a calm, secure place in which there is no room for ego.

While *Tokoyo* was under construction, my days were filled with both excitement and anxiety. There were so many obstacles I had to overcome. What would my family and neighbors think? "What is Masato up to now?" they would ask. I could put up with this criticism, but what about my family? Was I about to put them through another round of suffering? If I sat in front of Chisso every day, how could I make a living? I might even be arrested. Then what would happen to my family?

My biggest fear, however, was that I was embarking on a path of self-destruction. Once I stepped into the boat, would I just keep on rowing forever? A voice within me said even that would be all right. Since I had come this far, I couldn't turn back now. Once I had gone to Chisso as a victim, as a patient–activist; now I would go as an individual human being, as Ogata Masato.

At last *Tokoyo* was finished, and we held a boat-launching ceremony. It was May 1, 1987. It was a joyous occasion, exceeding all my expectations, and I was pleased to see many of my close friends.

The next morning I was awakened by a telephone call from Akazaki Satoru, who was then working at Minamata City Hall and serving on the city council. I was surprised. He had attended the boat launching, but this was the first time he had ever called me. When I picked up the receiver, Akazaki seemed relieved to hear my voice. In our local dialect, Akazaki said, "I was worried about you. Somehow I had the feeling that you were dying. I wasn't able to sleep at all. I just stayed awake waiting for dawn so that I could call you."

I was grateful for his concern. I told him that I too had been worried that when the boat was completed I would simply step in and keep rowing until I died. "But now that I've made it safely through the first night," I said, "I know I'm going to be OK." "You have a wife and precious daughters, so you've got to live for them," he replied. I was moved. From the kindness shown to me by everyone at the boat-launching ceremony, I learned that the call of this world was prevailing over the pull toward the other.

The invitation to live was stronger than the temptation to die.

The boat was ready, and I was determined to carry out my plan, but there

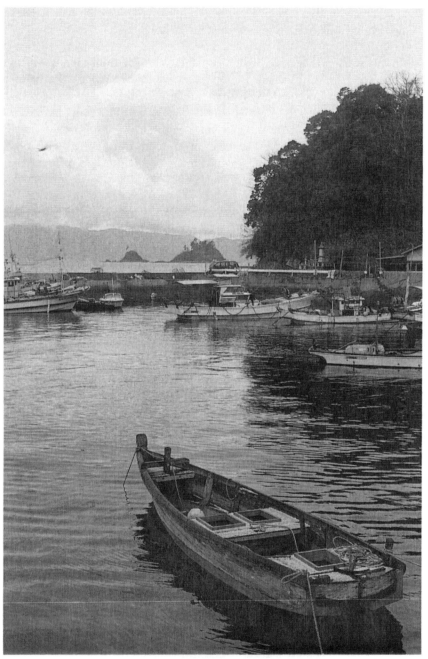

Tokoyo, moored at the pier in front of Masato's house

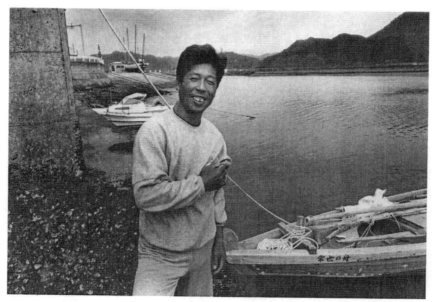

Masato with his new boat, Tokoyo, in 1987 (Photo by Akutagawa Jin)

were still a number of obstacles to overcome. First, I needed to see exactly how long it would take to sail to Minamata City. To go so far as to take a trial run, however, would be too calculating. It would be like taking out an insurance policy. I decided not to set off during the summer, in order to avoid hot, windless days. Winter would be ideal, when I could catch the northwesterly or easterly wind at dawn; the problem was the return. I wanted to sit in front of Chisso. But once I got settled, then what? Would people sneer and throw things at me? Would I be able to maintain my composure, to remain as calm as if I were at home?

Even if I had to postpone the trip, I felt it was important to deal with these questions one by one, by myself. If this had been a group undertaking, there would have been a division of labor. A group effort would have been quicker, but I was determined to do this by myself. I took my time and gave the matter a lot of thought. What was most important was to sit in front of Chisso, if only briefly, to expose my soul as a reminder of what they had done and of who I was. My very presence would serve as a mirror, exposing in turn the deeds and values of corporate Japan. If I made it safely through the first day of my sit-in, then I would make the trip early each week, weather permitting. There was no need to take any chances. I would be careful not to put my family through too much, while also looking out for my own health.

I didn't discuss all my doubts and questions with my wife; I simply told her my final decision. I'm not the type that consults with people. Once I've made up my mind, though, I'll take as long as necessary to help people understand my position. Perhaps because she knew there was no point in arguing, my wife accepted my decision. To tell you the truth, I was hoping she'd come along. But this was my own selfish desire, so I didn't mention it to her. If my wife had joined me on these journeys to Chisso, I would have been the happiest man in the world.

Bearing Witness

At last I was to embark on my maiden voyage. It was the seventh of December. If I had had to wait a day longer, I think I would have exploded. I cast off just before dawn, with my family waving from the beach. As I had expected, the wind was blowing from the east over the Shiranui Sea, sweeping the morning mist toward the Amakusa Islands. It promised to be a beautiful day. In the early light of dawn the *Eternal World* ran smoothly toward the south, catching the wind with its single sail. I was struck by the beautiful silhouette of the Ashikita Mountains with the sun still behind them. It was just as I was rounding Cape Daimon that the sun peeked over the hills.

Finally Minamata City came into view. I saw a cluster of gray factory buildings, their stacks emitting great clouds of smoke. In contrast to the idyllic shoreline fishing villages I had just passed, the Chisso complex was grotesque. As I drew closer, I could hear the sounds of the city and smell the sour, acidic odor of factory emissions.

Because they were in the midst of dredging operations to remove sludge contaminated with mercury in Marushima Port, I pulled in at the newly built dock close by. Fishermen and wholesalers at the morning market watched me in amazement. It seemed that they had forgotten that there had once been wooden rowing boats with sails.

I went to get a cart I had left near the dock several days earlier and loaded up my supplies, including a portable cooking stove, straw mats, and some *shochu*. I looked like a street vendor going off for a day's work. It was about a twenty-minute walk to the main gate of Chisso. I passed by the sluice gate, walked along a small path beside the factory canal, coming out on the national highway. It was about nine o'clock when I approached the factory gate. With my hands still on the cart handles, I paused to catch my breath. I wondered how many times I had imagined this moment. "I've come a long way," I heard myself say.

Chisso is surrounded by a canal, once used for waste water. Some might see it as a moat surrounding a castle. Through the canal runs a current of

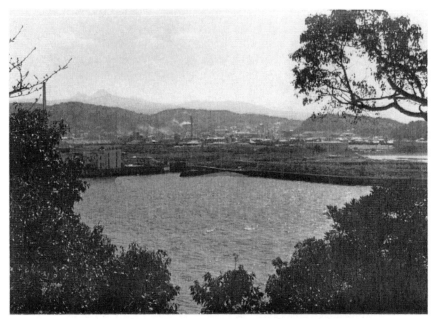

The Chisso factory complex, beyond the mouth of Minamata River

dark green slime. Just in front of the main gate is a bridge that crosses the canal. I parked my cart in the bicycle lot and crossed over the bridge to the guardhouse. "I'm Ogata from Meshima," I said. "I'm going to sit in front of the factory to make a statement about Minamata disease." The guard turned pale and dialed his supervisors.

Naturally, I hadn't warned Chisso of my visit, so it wasn't surprising that they were thrown off guard. Ignoring their confusion, I pulled a mat out of my cart and sat down in the bicycle parking lot. Before long, some company officials approached me saying, "Mr. Ogata, what is this all about?"

"I plan to sit here all day," I said.

"This is no place to talk," they said. "Come inside for a minute and we'll discuss this."

"There's no need to take me into the executive offices," I replied. "I'm fine right here, so don't go to any trouble."

It was laughable. "Discuss," indeed. Where had they been all these years when we wanted to talk to them? At present I had no intention of discussing anything. We would exhaust the words in the language before we could bridge the gap between us. This was the main gate, Chisso's public face, and they had no idea what I had in mind. "I'm not here to disrupt your business," I assured them. This was true.

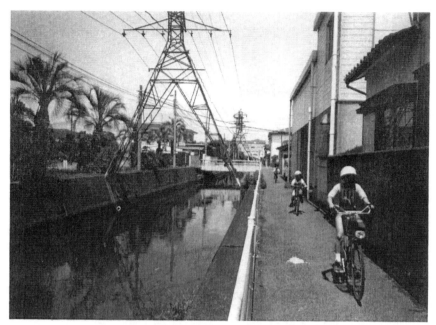

A canal borders the Chisso factory (left). The bridge in the center leads to the main gate of the factory.

Soon I pulled out some more straw mats and began writing appeals, using black and red paint. The appeals were directed to three parties: the employees of Chisso, the victims, and the general public. I had planned to do this in advance, but I thought it important that the content of the message come right from my heart, dictated by the time and place. I couldn't complete them all in one day; I would finish the work when I returned. When the messages were complete, I stood the mats up behind me against a chain-link fence. In front of the mats I placed a framed photograph of my father. These are my messages. [The capitalized phrases were written in red. All of the messages were written in local dialect.]

To the employees of Chisso:
The Minamata Incident began when people stopped seeing their fellow humans as human beings. Isn't it time for you to accept your BASIC RESPONSIBILITIES AS HUMAN BEINGS? Somehow, please, please respond to this open letter. You, the folks at Chisso, COME BACK SOON. COME HOME!

To THOSE WHO HAVE SUFFERED:
Minamata disease has been absorbed by the system. All you hear nowadays is talk of lawsuits and official certification. Hey, wake up! Doesn't this mean that you are

being controlled by the state and the prefecture? What is Minamata disease really about? It's about the way we live. We need to live in harmony with the ocean and hills around us. We are NOT VICTIMS! We must live as HUMANS!

To the General Public:
Just imagine. The national government plans to stage an environmental exposition in Minamata. The same people who killed us like insects will now stage this farce, as if to draw the curtain on Minamata disease. Respectable citizens, WILL YOU STILL CONTINUE TO IGNORE WHAT IS HAPPENING?

The day brought many unexpected responses. First of all, a policeman stopped to see me. It wasn't that he had been summoned; he just happened to be doing his rounds on a bicycle. We talked for about thirty minutes. He told me it hadn't been more than a few months since he was transferred from the Amakusa Islands. He looked about fifty. "Where are you from?" he asked, and "What is it that you want?" He didn't seem to have any objections to my being there; he simply asked these questions out of general curiosity. He assumed that I was there representing an organization. When I said I'd come on my own, he was astonished. When I added that I wasn't making any demands, he looked even more surprised. He read through my straw-mat statements, slowly and thoughtfully. And what do you think he said as he

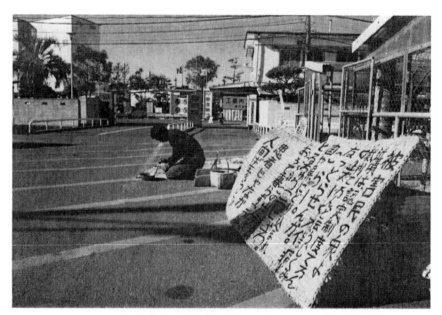

Masato writes a message on a straw mat during his one-man sit-in before the front gate of the Chisso factory. The message on the straw mat to his left encourages Minamata disease sufferers to live as humans, not as victims (December 1987).

left? "Hang in there!" Now it was my turn to be surprised. Before I made the trip I had braced myself against the possibility of being arrested.

As I began cooking some fish over my small charcoal stove, my first visitor was a cat. I gave him a bit of fish and he stayed with me for over an hour. I was moved by his respectful and compassionate attitude. I was so happy that tears came to my eyes. I realized how lonely I had been and for how long I had suppressed my feelings. The cat must have sensed these feelings. Usually when you feed a stray cat it grabs the food and runs. It doesn't stay around to visit.

After several trips I became pretty proficient at rowing and sailing to Minamata. If all went well, it took about two and a half hours from my house to Marushima Harbor. But I was still aware that anything could happen, depending on the weather and the direction of the wind. Winter weather was especially unpredictable, so it was important not to take any chances. Rather than adhere to a rigid schedule, I would pick my days according to the weather and the way I felt. When the weather continued to be bad, I would forget about the boat and take the bus. On an average day I would leave the house at dawn and arrive at Chisso's main gate around nine. After seeing all the workers off at the end of the day, I would load up my cart and begin the journey home around six.

There were many types of people who stopped by to chat with me as I sat before Chisso, and I enjoyed each one of them. Newspaper reporters and broadcast journalists would drop by and ask, "How long do you plan to continue doing this?" A schedule had never entered my mind. Just to please them, I would answer, "Until I'm tired of sitting." Supporters came to encourage me, but people I'd never met before would also stop by. One guy on his way to a hot spring read my messages and said, "I'd like to support your cause." "Your warm thoughts are quite enough," I answered. After all, this wasn't costing me anything. There were also people who dropped by with *mikan* and pastries. Some even brought letters of support.

I learned a great deal from children. It was children stopping by on their way home from school who proved to be the most serious readers of my straw-mat messages. I hadn't considered that children would think about these things. So, right away, I wrote a message on a white cloth especially for them and hung it on the fence.

> To the children:
> This happened when I was six.
> My father died of Minamata disease.
> Because of Chisso's poison, his hands and his legs shook.
> He could no longer stand and walk.
> He drooled, went into fits of madness, and finally died.
> After that the other children teased me, calling me
> "Minamata disease kid." They threw stones at me.

Their cruelty caused as much suffering as the disease.
Now, everyone,
PLEASE THINK HARD ABOUT MINAMATA DISEASE!
This incident has something very important to teach us.

Most of the workers going in and out of the factory would just pass by, glancing at me out of the corner of their eyes. But among them were a few who would greet me and take the time to read the straw-mat messages. I enjoyed watching their reactions. I was interested to note that the same person might have different attitudes, depending on the circumstances. A man might greet me cheerfully when he came out the factory alone, but if he was with his fellow workers, he wouldn't look my way. I could see the way peer pressure controlled their actions. When I drank *shochu*, I invited passers-by to join me. Although most of the men declined, saying, "I'm still at work," I felt some warmth in their response. When I was weaving a pair of traditional sandals called *ashinaka*, a Chisso worker came by and took a great interest in what I was doing. He said he would love to have a pair like that, so I made him some. He was delighted.

I didn't know how to make these sandals before I began my sit-in, but I thought it would be a good way to pass the time, so I began learning from my mother-in-law. They aren't easy to make! At first I couldn't make a matched pair—the shape and the size of each sandal were different. Finally, after many attempts, I created two sandals that could pass for a matched pair.

Once I started sandal weaving, people would look on with a nostalgic air. One old man picked up a sandal and said, "When I was young, this was all we wore." An old woman stopped by to give me advice on improving my technique. I loved to watch their expressions as they drifted back to the old days. Those stony faces that had been watching for the light to change had suddenly softened. Even a Chisso worker would, for a moment, lose his company face when he picked up a sandal, sighing, "These bring back memories."

About a month after my sit-in began, I could see tension building among the Chisso executives. Public-security officers came around to check out what I was doing. But in the end the company decided not to force me from my spot. They probably didn't want to stir up media attention. When they learned that I was simply sitting there by myself, not interfering with traffic, not using a loudspeaker to agitate workers, and not disturbing company operations, they figured it was best to leave me alone. But they didn't like it. I wouldn't like it either if some strange man appeared in front of my house and began cooking his fish and drinking *shochu*. It seems that at first they thought I would be there for one day only, but I kept coming back every week. Then they knew I was serious, but—and I think this is very important—they couldn't for the life of them figure out my purpose in being there. Each worker seemed to interpret my intentions in a different way.

Some people came up and said, "What do you hope to gain from this, anyway?" Or, "You aren't going to be able to communicate anything to them in this way." They were missing the point. From the beginning, I had nothing to gain and nothing to demand. This is exactly what I wanted to show them. I simply want to live one day at a time sitting in front of Chisso, bearing witness to what they had done and to what they now represented. How they chose to interpret my actions was up to them. I threw a stone into the pond, but the ripples were not my concern.

Toward the end of April a Chisso worker approached me and asked, "Would you mind if we string up carp streamers?" He was very apologetic, and without waiting for my answer he went on to explain, "We have no intention of interfering with what you are doing, but this is an annual custom. Please understand." I couldn't believe that they would think I had objections to putting up decorations for Boy's Day on May 5. I simply replied that it would be no problem. The worker seemed much relieved and returned with a long pole, onto which he hoisted the streamers. I loved watching the colorful carp, swaying and swimming through the breeze above my head. I wished that I could be as light and carefree.

As I mentioned before, I hadn't thought about how long I would continue my sit-in. But eventually I felt that the time to quit was drawing near. In May the sun was already high, making it hot and uncomfortable. The asphalt was like a furnace. The heat made me dizzy. Finally I decided that to force myself to continue, neglecting my physical condition, would only invite serious problems. If I forced the issue, I would end up relying on other people for help and blaming them when things went wrong. So I decided to bring my sit-in to a close at the end of May.

Before I left, I had an opportunity to tour the Chisso factory. It was something I had long wanted to do, and so I put in a request. During my days in the movement I had been in the conference room, but I had never visited the factory itself. I had no idea exactly where the mercury had been used and discarded. I assume that other activists had never been in the plant either. It seems strange that those most concerned did not try to create the opportunity to look at the factory firsthand.

The company agreed, and on the arranged day I took my wife and three daughters to Minamata. The company provided two cars and gave us a splendid guided tour. Apparently the focus of production at that time was chemical fertilizers and photographic film. Our visit took place on a Saturday, when the factory was not in operation. Just for us, they conducted an experiment in the building where liquid nitrogen and liquid oxygen were stored. At the end of the tour they gave each of my girls a notebook and pencil, and they presented my wife and me each with a card-sized calculator with a crystal screen. Chisso had been one of the innovators in liquid crystal technol-

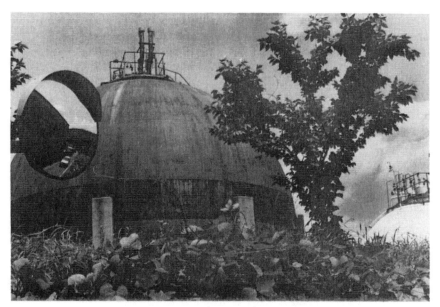

A process vessel in the Chisso compound

ogy. They were treating us so well, it was almost overbearing. Although I feel that they were sincere in their own way, it was a little hard for me to accept.

When I informed Chisso of my decision to end the sit-in at the end of May, they looked relieved and said, "To tell you the truth, Mr. Ogata, we didn't know what to make of this." Until I came, all of the sit-ins had been conducted by groups, and their demands had been quite predictable. In my case, however, they didn't understand what I wanted, so they couldn't think of any way to respond. They were simply cogs in a machine, they told me. If they had responded to me with any kind of initiative or imagination, they would have been replaced immediately.

It was then that the officials invited me to a dinner. I declined. They insisted that they had no ulterior motives, but I felt that once this got out there would be serious misunderstandings. Later on in June they phoned again. This time they said they wanted to treat my children to a meal. I couldn't find any reason to refuse when the invitation was extended to my whole family, so I agreed that we would meet them in the town of Sashiki.

Soon after that, my daughter Mamiko drowned in the ocean. I still don't know how to handle my emotions; this isn't something I can talk about. I can say, though, that I'm glad I took her to see Chisso before she passed away. There is no way to overcome the emptiness, but I cherish the memories of her coming out to the beach to see me off each time I headed for Minamata.

A Will of Stone

Early in 1990 I learned that the governor of Kumamoto, Hosokawa Morihiro, was planning to hold a concert on the land reclaimed by filling the polluted seabed of Minamata Bay. This is the same Hosokawa who would later become prime minister of Japan. The event was to be called "Concert for Ten Thousand People," and it would commemorate the supposed resurrection of the environment and reconstruction of the community of Minamata. I couldn't believe it. How dare they stage a party on a site symbolic of so many years of suffering? This wasn't the kind of place to have a raucous gathering. I decided to speak directly to the governor. When I told my wife, she said that this time she would accompany me. She must have realized how lonely I was each time I set out in my boat for Minamata. I was so happy. To have her at my side was better than having a million people behind me. That is why the letter I submitted to the governor and to the mayor of Minamata contains both of our signatures.

First I called the governor's office and asked for a meeting so we could discuss some issues related to the reclaimed land. I was told that the governor's schedule was so tight that it would be impossible but that they could arrange a meeting with the vice governor. The date was set for July 1. At the end of June, I received a call from the section chief of the Planning Department. He said he wanted to come and talk to me. I said I didn't see the need, but he insisted. I happened to have some business coming up in Sashiki, so I told him I would meet him at the prefectural office building there. He asked me exactly why I wanted to speak with the vice governor. "I simply want to discuss something with him," I replied. The section chief left without getting any information from me.

On the scheduled day, my wife and I went to Kumamoto City. When we arrived at the Prefectural Hall, several reporters were waiting for me. I had told the vice governor's office that I wanted our meeting to be public, and I had contacted the journalists myself. Since we were early, we all decided to go to a coffee shop and wait. But when our appointment time came around,

117

no one called us in. "We didn't know the media would be present," they told
me. "I didn't come here to hold a private conversation," I reminded them.
"I told you that this was to be public." Another hour passed before we were
invited in. The vice governor sent out a message that he would like me to
get rid of the journalists. "There's no reason to do so," I said. "I have nothing
to hide. But if you want to use this as an excuse not to meet with me, I'll
show up at your house with my wife and kids and enough provisions to camp
out for a while." The vice governor agreed that we had better meet now.

The meeting lasted for about an hour. I handed my letter to the vice governor and then explained my position further. The meeting ended with a
brief question-and-answer session with the press. The vice governor seemed
to be listening seriously throughout. This is the text of my letter:

> There is a conspiracy at work to deny the very existence of Minamata disease. We
> see this in the development plans for the reclaimed land of Minamata Bay. The
> conspirators are the state and its agents.
>
> We will not tolerate this course of action. We stand together to beat down your
> plans. It is clear that your development project is nothing more than an attempt to
> hide the scene of the crime. You hide under such slogans as "environmental restora-
> tion" and all your talk about a memorial tower and facilities for tourism and recre-
> ation. Your real intent is to encourage people to forget about Minamata disease. You
> are ready to waste fifteen billion yen on this project, and then you hope to make a
> profit from it. We are appalled by your lack of respect. To continue with these plans
> will certainly invite divine punishment. We demand that you drop this project
> immediately.
>
> At the same time, we would like to ask the general public, "Are we going to
> repeat the same mistake?" We turn our ear toward the Shiranui Sea, praying for a
> more enlightened state of mind. The reclaimed land is the grave of all those who
> died in this Sea of Sorrow. Are we to disturb these souls once again? This is the
> grave of Minamata disease. Let us leave a place for it, both here on land and in the
> annals of history.
>
> In prayer,
Ogata Masato
Ogata Sawako

Normally top officials don't accommodate individual requests for meetings. I was a familiar face in that office, however, and they probably didn't
want to deal with the consequences of refusing. My wife admitted later that
she didn't believe the vice governor would actually meet with us. It also
seemed strange to her that the officials seemed so uncomfortable with our
presence. She had never been in a government office, and everything was
new to her.

For me, one of the greatest successes of the meeting was having my wife at my side. Although I found it a little bit embarrassing at first, ultimately her presence made me feel more powerful. When you take some action on your own, the government will assume that it's a matter of personal ideology and may ignore it as irrelevant. However, when a couple or a whole family act together, it's hard for officials to dismiss them summarily. A family is something they can relate to. They may see that the family's request is a matter of daily survival, not simply personal philosophy. Most Japanese see government officials like the governor and vice governor as figures beyond their reach. They should learn that if they have the will, even common fisherfolk like ourselves can gain access to these people.

In the end, the "Concert for Ten Thousand People" was held. The weather was good that morning, but by the afternoon a thunderstorm was brewing. Suddenly it began to pour. Most of the two to three thousand people attending the concert had been recruited by the government from various schools and institutions. As the storm picked up, they began to run. The event was a disaster. I had been standing at the entrance, distributing pamphlets protesting the event. The storm exceeded my wildest dreams. "It's the fury of our local gods," I said to a friend.

In September, Governor Hosokawa declared that no further large-scale events would be held on the reclaimed land. He soon resigned as governor. As you know, he reappeared on the political stage as prime minister, but he didn't last too long there either. There must have been many reasons for his resigning as governor of Kumamoto, but I would like to believe that the disastrous concert was among them.

From the outset, I had opposed filling in the bay. This opinion was shared by many, and the reclamation project even became the focus of a court battle. In the end, though, we lost, and fifty-eight hectares of bay were filled. On the inland side of the reclaimed land you can see the Chisso plant, a canal for wastewater, and a sluice box through which the company is believed to have emptied huge quantities of toxicants. On the opposite side lies the ocean; close at hand you see Koiji Island.

After Hosokawa abandoned Kumamoto for Tokyo, plans for developing the land went through a series of changes. The latest plan is to develop a greenbelt of fields and woods. I don't think this is a bad idea. But what is most important to me is the way we feel when we stand on this sacred spot. If we forget this element, all the arguments over land use become meaningless. People often clamor for their "rights," for which the Japanese word is *ken-ri*. But after you've repeated "*ken-ri*" a number of times, it becomes indistinguishable from another Japanese word, *ri-ken*. This means "one's vested interests" or "money grabbing." Along with our rights to develop and forget, let us not neglect our responsibilities to preserve and remember.

A Place of Atonement

The reclaimed land in Minamata Bay illustrates the laws of karma. It demonstrates more clearly than any other place I've seen the relationship between cause and effect. Looking at the original topography of this region, we see first the ocean, then the tidelands. Hills lead into the mountains. Mountain forests are the source of our fresh water, which flows back down to the sea. Land and ocean are intimately connected. Here at the reclaimed land these natural links have been severed by concrete barriers and terraces. The reclaimed land is highly symbolic. It reminds us that Minamata disease represents the destruction of natural cycles.

Originally everything was returned to the ocean. But this is no longer possible. In our greed we have created things that cannot be returned safely to the earth and the sea. The accumulation of toxic sediments in Minamata Bay is similar to the problem of nuclear waste disposal. At a loss for how to dispose of it, we bury it with soil and go on with our business.

On paper the reclaimed land belongs to Kumamoto Prefecture, but because the national government was also involved in the landfill project, it too has a say in its use. However, I'd like to ask them to relinquish their claims. This is a place that should not be owned by anyone. Fundamentally, what does land ownership mean? Ownership should entail stewardship—stewardship that continues from one generation to the next. One lifetime is too short to exercise ownership.

Minamata Bay has been called the source of Minamata disease. Each one of us must confront this place in his own way. For me, it is a place of atonement. It is a place to contemplate my own guilt and to offer my own apology.

In 1993, a group of us began talking about placing Buddhist statues, *nobotoke*, on the reclaimed land. *Nobotoke* are small stone images of the kind you will find along the roadside and at crossroads in rural areas. After several meetings we decided to go ahead with the idea, and in the spring of the following year seventeen Minamata disease patients got together to compose a "A Statement of Original Vow." In Japanese *hongan*, or "original vow," refers to our deepest wish, our most fervent prayer. I wrote the first draft. This is how it begins:

> Once Minamata Bay was the treasure chest of our sea. Here schools of fish came to spawn. The young fry matured here and then returned to repeat the cycle. The bay was like a womb. In what is now landfill between Hyakken Port and Myojin Point, the silver scales of sardine and gizzard shad shimmered in the sunlight. Mullet leapt. Shrimp and crab frolicked in the shallows. At low tide we collected shellfish. At the edge of the waves we gathered seaweed—*wakame* and *hijiki*. These were the things that nourished us.

This natural wealth was destroyed by industrial civilization. In our statement I refer to this tragedy that is repeated through human history as man's "original sin." If Minamata Bay and its landfill symbolize the depth of human sin, then this ought also to be a place where humans can acknowledge their sin, atone for it, and pray. This is why I welcomed the idea of placing *nobotoke* at this spot. The statement ends with these words:

> On this land reclaimed from the Sea of Sorrow, we vow to enshrine small stone images. Bowing down before them, we will clasp our hands in prayer, contemplate the sins of man, and pray for the salvation of those souls lost to organic mercury. It is our deepest wish that this land of disease and death be transformed into a Pure Land of the spirit, where all creatures may be consoled.

—March 2, 1994
Concerned Minamata Disease Patients

The carving and placing of each image will be a highly personal act. Each image will represent my apologies and prayers; it will be a substitute for this body of flesh. The images will also serve as intermediaries through whom we may communicate with the souls of the deceased. A reunification of the living and dead is our greatest wish, our most fervent prayer.

Hongan no Kai, the Association of Original Vow, held its first meeting on January 29, 1995, in Minamata City. It's not exactly an organization but an informal gathering of individuals with different opinions and positions. The only belief we shared at the beginning was that there could be no such thing as a "total" or "final" solution to the Minamata disease incident. Since then we have been working slowly to carve our statues, plant trees, and gradually restore the hills and sea to their natural state.

In June of that year I took a trip to Okinawa. I had some wonderful opportunities. I was able to meet musician Kina Shokichi, whose music and social activism had long inspired me. Ethnographic photographer Higa Yasuo, who has spent years documenting traditional rituals and ceremonies of the Okinawan islands, kindly took me to many of the *utaki*, sacred places, on the Miyako Islands. As I think about our *nobotoke* and ponder the possibility of a spiritual homeland, the spiritual traditions of Okinawa often come to mind.

At the end of July, Kina came to Minamata with his group, "Champloose," and gave a concert on the reclaimed land. Kina was on his way to Hiroshima and Nagasaki to perform in commemoration of the fiftieth anniversary of the atomic bomb. The group had set off from the westernmost island of Okinawa in a traditional wooden canoe called a *sabani*.

The concert was so much fun that I found myself dancing. I heard some-one complain that the man who had fought against the governor's concert was now staging his own on the same ground. I dismissed this by saying sim-ply, "It's OK if it's me." I was only half-joking.

The concert took place on the shore, looking out on Koiji Island. Due to the landfill this small island is now so close to shore that you can hear cicadas singing in its woods. At one time the island was used as a leper colony. For some time, though, it has been uninhabited, and nature has been free to take its course without human interference. It was only because of the Minamata incident that developers kept their distance, and so, ironically, we find today a bit of old-growth forest right next to a city. For decades this island has been a silent witness to the development of the Minamata region. In my view Koiji Island is a sacred place. We must leave it untouched as a measure of what we have lost.

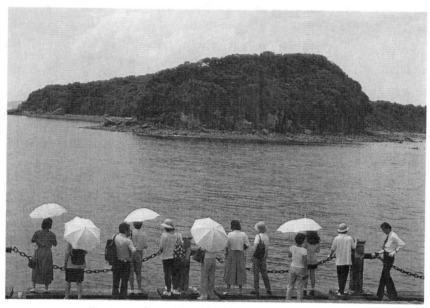

Tourists on the reclaimed land look toward Koiji Island.

Before the land reclamation took place, there was a spit that jutted out toward Koiji Island. It is believed that this is where, in ancient times, the first inhabitants of our region stepped out of their canoes after the long voyage from the southern islands. Looking at this story as both history and myth, we may also see this as a place where gods descended. Walking through the woods here recently I found an ancient place of prayer, reminding me of sacred sites in Okinawa. Around a pair of giant *akou*, a kind of banyan tree, are the remnants of a stagelike structure made from large boulders. Today the tree roots have worked their way between and around the stones, embracing their secrets. It seems a miracle that this one patch of woods on a small knoll remains as it was, overlooking a plain of landfill.

Developers are now taking a close look at this region. I even heard about a plan to build a bridge from the reclaimed land to Koiji Island. There seems to be no end to greed in the human heart. Just wait and see. Soon we'll hear demands for improving the reclaimed land with vending machines, toilets, telephone booths, and parking lots. If we just sit back and let it happen, our sacred places will disappear before our eyes. We must protect these remaining patches of forest. They will help us reconnect with the natural world. Our woods and our small stone images will serve as our guides, leading us on a path of healing and restoration.

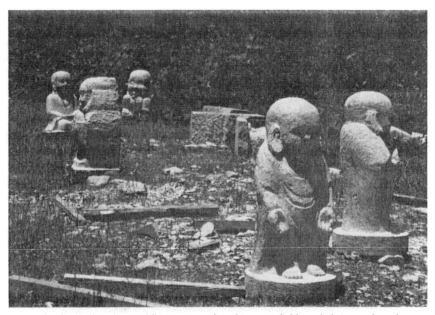

Unfinished nobotoke, *Buddhist statues placed in open fields and along rural roads, carved by the members of Hongan-no-kai*

TRANSLATOR'S NOTES

1. On May 22, 1973, a Kumamoto University research team reported a possible third outbreak of Minamata disease along the west coast of the Ariake Sea, forty kilometers north of Minamata. (The first outbreak occurred in Minamata City in 1956 and the second in Niigata in 1965.) This third outbreak allegedly resulted from effluent dumped by the Nippon Synthetic Chemical Industry. In June 1973, consumer anxiety about mercury in fish and shellfish increased when high concentrations of mercury were found along the beach in front of the Tokuyama Soda Plant in Tokuyama, Yamaguchi Prefecture. In 1974, the Environment Agency declined to recognize Minamata disease victims in either region. Iijima Mobuko, ed., *Pollution Japan: Historical Chronology* (Tokyo: Asahi Evening News, 1979), 350, 354; Kurihara Akira, *Shogen Minamato byo* (Tokyo: Iwanami Shoten, 2000); *Minamata byo kanren nenpyo*, 4.

2. The Kanemi Corporation heated its cooking oil to 210–230 degrees Centigrade in the deodorizing stage by passing polychlorinated biphenyls (PCBs) through stainless-steel pipes in the oil vats. In February 1968, pipes in a newly installed vat in the Kitakyushu plant overheated, developing pinhole-sized openings that allowed PCBs to enter the vegetable oil. Victims of the incident appeared in twenty-three prefectures. In addition to pitting and discoloration of the skin, PCB poisoning causes cysts, pain in the joints, secretions from the eyes, and respiratory, bone, and liver disorders. Ariyoshi Sawako, *Fukugo osen* (Compound Pollution), 2 vols. (Tokyo: Shinchosha, 1975) 2: 127–38; Norie Huddle and Michael Reich, *Island of Dreams: Environmental Crisis in Japan* (New York: Autumn, 1975), 133–44.

3. The Burakumin, or Buraku people, are descendents of a group of Japanese involved, from the eighth century, in such occupations as disposing of dead people, killing animals, and doing leatherwork. Contact with blood and death were considered defilements in early Japanese Shinto society, and the killing of animals was a sin according to Buddhist precepts. The Tokugawa shogunate (1600–1868) took advantage of these religious strictures to place the Burakumin at the lowest rung of society, together with convicted criminals and other "nonpeople." The symbolic status of the untouchable emperor at the top and the untouchable Burakumin at the bottom served well the interests of military rule. Stigmas inherited from the past continue to cloud the lives of Burakumin descendants.

Part Three

常世の舟

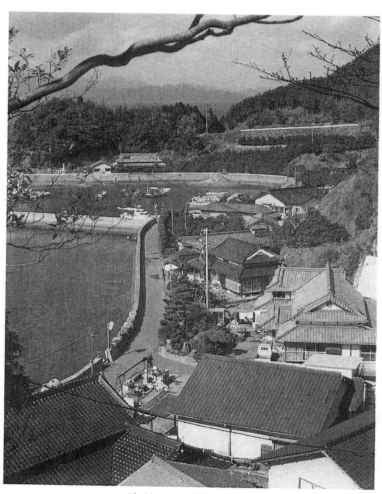

The hamlet of Ikenoshiri

Beneath the Light of the Sun and the Moon

In September 1999, our region was hit by a great typhoon. The winds tore the roofs right off many houses, and the typhoon left extensive damage in other ways as well. It was the strongest typhoon in my memory. Fortunately, my house was not damaged, but I was left with a deep impression of the ferocity with which nature can unleash her power. Most of the trees we had planted along the water on the reclaimed land were ripped from the earth, roots and all. Only the small stone Buddhas we had chiseled from large pieces of rock remained standing among the fallen trees. They continued to gaze tranquilly out toward Koiji Island and the sea beyond.

There are about thirty stone Buddhas along the beach. I'm chiseling my third one right now. I'm not very skillful, but I enjoy the process. Taking advantage of bits of spare time in my daily life, I chisel the stone slowly and deliberately, as if imbuing it with my own flesh and blood. I will give this project as much time as it needs; the piece will let me know when it is done. It feels good to entrust myself to the flow of time, devoting body and soul to my work.

I look upon these stone Buddhas as a kind of relay station. They make it possible for us to communicate with the spirits of the deceased, be they people, fish, birds, or cats. There is a growing tendency in Japan today for people to negate the past or to twist events around so they can be justified. Expressions such as "aiming for the future" and "looking ahead" have become popular, but we should realize that underlying these expressions is our intent to "settle the accounts of the past." The political settlement of the Minamata disease issue falls into this category. It is my belief that to negate the past is to negate the future. It is precisely because of its links to the past that the future becomes possible. The past is part of my being that has no end. I continue to live tied to the souls of those who have passed on.

This reminds me of a dialogue that took place in 1995, on the fiftieth anniversary of the end of World War II. Politicians and bureaucrats alike staged farcical debates about whether Japan should apologize to countries

129

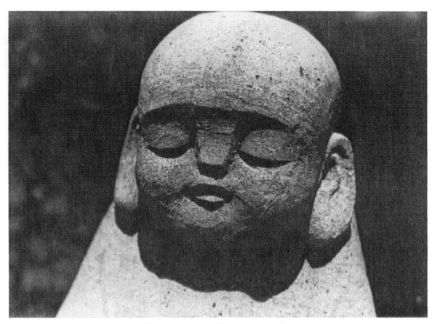

Stone statues carved by members of Hongan-no-kai face the ocean on land reclaimed from Minamata Bay

that suffered from Japan's wartime aggression and domination, and what the wording for such apologies should be, were they to be tendered. That same autumn it became clear that the various factions of Minamata disease victims were willing, at last, to accept a "final resolution" in the form of a compromise position offered by the government. Once again we were ready to "settle the accounts" of a dark past.

It was around that time that I left for Europe. My traveling companions were a staff member from Soshisha and two professors from Kumamoto University. All three had participated in some way in the Minamata struggle. Even before they invited me to join them, I had long wished to visit Germany and Poland. I wanted to see the relics of the Nazi concentration camps. The word "Auschwitz" resonated strongly in my soul. I wanted to see this place and to find my own place within it. We spent a month in Germany and Poland. Such a long trip was a first for me. I walked long distances. I hadn't realized I possessed such stamina. My self-confidence grew.

The concentration camps were more horrible than I had dared to imagine. I had heard about the gas chambers, but I learned that the Nazis had showed no lack of creativity in their methods of killing. Some Jews had been poi-

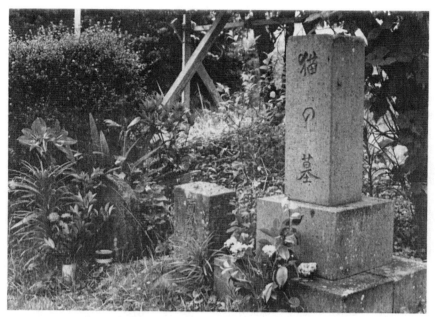

Neko-no-haka, *a grave for cats that died of Minamata disease,
in the garden of Soshisha, Minamata City*

soned. Others had been shot. As I gazed at prisoners' fingernails left in an underground chamber, I felt the room fill with screams and cries of despair.

After I had visited a number of these sites, a question took form in my mind. "If I had been living in Germany during Hitler's regime, what would I have done?" Before the trip to Germany I had already asked myself on several occasions, "What stance would I have taken toward Minamata disease had I been an employee of Chisso?" This new question bore down on me even more heavily. Why had this totalitarian way of thinking spread so quickly? Why had the general populace not only embraced this ideology but supported it with such zeal? Why wasn't that precept of mercy, at the heart of most religions, able to check the brutality of Nazi actions? Why was there so little resistance?

Generally, when people speak of the Holocaust, they are satisfied with the explanation that the Nazis were responsible and that this horrific bit of history grew out of Hitler's insanity. This is no different from saying that Japan's role in World War II was the responsibility of state militarism and the emperor system. This is certainly one interpretation, but if we stop there we fail to acknowledge the responsibility each one of us should bear for supporting the Nazis or the emperor system.

Before talking about the responsibility that should be borne by Chisso or the state for Minamata disease, I had taken it upon myself to consider my own sins, my own responsibility for this incident. Now I wanted to know how Germans felt about and dealt with one of the most heinous crimes in human history. On whom did Germans place the responsibility for these crimes? What did the past mean to them, and how did it relate to their future? How was the older generation passing down their experiences to the younger, if at all?

There was no reason to expect a clear answer to these questions during a short visit. But I received any number of hints. I learned that children all study the Holocaust as part of their school curriculum. I learned that the Germans are actively pursuing the issue of war crimes. It became clear that the Germans plan to preserve the camps so that these crimes will continue to be exposed to future generations. Standing in stark contrast was Japan's attitude that our country's crimes must be covered up and erased from memory. Some people say that Germany takes this position because it is highly sensitive to the critical eyes of the countries that surround it. The Japanese state, on the other hand, is indifferent to other Asian countries. But it is oversensitive to American opinion.

I think that what prompted me to go to Europe was the desire to verify my own humanity. It's dangerous not to do this now and then. We can degenerate before we know it. Human beings are weak. It was, after all, the average person who embraced Nazi ideology and worshipped Hitler. Can any of us say with certainty that this would never happen to us? It was the average person who betrayed family members and turned in friends, informing on those who had even the slightest bit of Jewish blood from distant ancestors. Homosexuals and the physically handicapped received the same treatment as the Jews.

Before I went to Europe I saw the movie *Schindler's List*. As I traveled I thought a lot about this man. I'm fascinated by people like Schindler who are able to take action on their own initiative. Some of the most powerful forces in human history are unleashed not by the teachings or ideologies of a system or group but by those of a rather self-centered individual. Although the average man was swept up by Nazi ideology, Schindler, another average man, was able to reverse course. Rather than giving in to the system, he followed his own beliefs.

While traveling in Germany we had the opportunity to attend a conference on environmental technology convened by Japanese and German scholars. Most of the participants were economists, sociologists, engineers, and so on. The conference was sponsored by the Japanese embassy and Japanese companies based in Germany, so their representatives spoke as well. There was simultaneous interpretation, and all in all, it appeared to be a very costly meeting. Most of the talks were of a technical nature, not venturing beyond the parameters of their authors' own scholarly fields. Most centered on the fanciful theme of "harmonious development," advocating the idea that environmental problems could be eliminated by technology. The general mood was upbeat.

Since the four of us had all lived through the Minamata crisis, we felt, quite naturally, that something was wrong with this sort of reasoning. We thought that what needed to be discussed was not a technological revolution but a transformation of our basic values. I heard that East Germany had become a dumping ground for the West. It had even been polluted with mercury waste. I asked several of the conference participants what they thought about the disappearance of fish from the rivers. They went blank and could not respond. It seemed that they had never given any thought to the matter. Perhaps it had never entered their minds that some time in the past people had fished those rivers and eaten the fish. Pollution is a problem. But the myth that these problems can be overcome with technology alone is an even greater problem.

Three men who represented corporations that did business in Germany came forward to participate in a panel discussion. One of these companies was Showa Denko—the very same Showa Denko that was responsible for Minamata disease in Niigata. I listened intently to catch what its speaker might have to say about Minamata disease, but he never touched upon the subject. According to this speaker, three parties had been cooperating closely until the present—industry, the government, and academia. He said that it was necessary now to add a fourth element—the local resident. The cooperation of these four groups would ensure that everything ran smoothly, he concluded. I was shocked that he didn't say a word about Minamata disease, and his condescending attitude as a conference sponsor irked me.

I decided to stand up and speak my mind. First, I introduced myself as a victim of Minamata disease. Even if he had expected a participant from Minamata, he certainly did not expect to confront a victim. The auditorium became absolutely silent. The speaker's face paled. "I have no intention of blaming you personally for Minamata disease," I began. "But I'd like to know why, in your speech today, you didn't say one word about this incident." Realizing that there would be people present who considered Minamata disease to be an event of the past, I decided to explain further. Even now, thirty years later, victims are suffering while the question of responsibility remains contested, I said. The recent compromise position crafted by the government had created a great stir throughout the country, I went on, but Showa Denko was not part of this settlement, and people were waiting for the company's response. How, in the midst of this commotion, could a representative of this company pretend that Minamata had never happened and blithely talk about solving environmental problems? What kind of cooperation did Showa Denko seek from the residents to whom they had caused such suffering? Was this so-called cooperation between industry, government, academia, and local residents based on equally distributed power? What did cooperation mean to a company that had just poisoned local residents? How could there be a future for a company that would not own up to its past?

The speaker from Showa Denko hung his head in silence. It was as if he'd been ambushed. During the coffee break, people flooded to my side saying they had been moved or impressed by what I had said. Even people who had ignored me before, because I had neither business card nor title, now came to greet me.

Months before the trip to Europe, I had begun to consider walking from my home to Minamata City, but I had entertained doubts about my strength. Now, after walking through Germany and Poland, I had gained confidence. Of course, I did get a boost from the wonderful local wine and beer there!

I decided that my destination now, back in Japan, would be the reclaimed land in Minamata. Metaphorically speaking, that reclaimed-land site was, in the geography of my small universe, another Auschwitz. It was my personal Auschwitz, a place where life had been poisoned, a prison where one could still hear the cries of the deceased. I would start walking toward that spot.

Walking. That was something to which I could entrust my entire body and soul. Generally we speak of entrusting ourselves to the state, or to society, or to the times, but that is dangerous. I wanted to entrust myself to the mountains and sea of the place I was born. As I walked, I would empty my mind. I wanted to feel myself as one with the mountains and sea. These were my thoughts.

On New Year's Day, 1996, I left my house before sunrise. In my hands I held a walking stick. On my back was a rucksack. A puppy was my companion. I had rescued the dog from the pound, thereby saving it from the fate of being fed to lions and tigers at the zoo. Why did I decide to take the dog? I guess it was because I thought I would be lonely. It was important to me that the dog and I could communicate only through exchanges of feelings. There would be no words, leading to arguments and theories. However, as we went along, I found that the young dog tired long before I did. When the sun rose and cars began zooming past, I had to be careful that the dog didn't run out into the road. As we approached the city, local dogs began to bark at him. In the end, he was more trouble than he was worth.

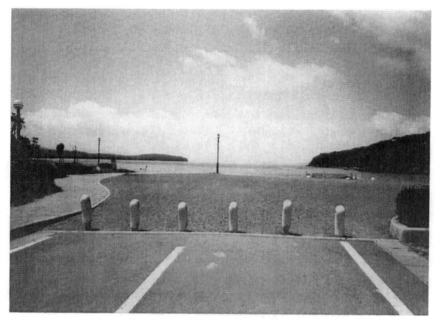

This road ends where the reclaimed land meets the sea.

Avoiding the highway, I followed the coastal route, winding between the mountains and sea. It took about six hours, including rest stops, to reach Minamata City. As I approached the Chisso factory, I heard a siren announce noon break. By the time I reached the reclaimed land, my legs and hips were stressed to the limit, and once I had settled down, I couldn't get up again. I ate the rice balls I had brought for lunch, downed some *shochu*, and fell into a deep sleep.

Everything in our current industrial society moves at such high speed that we are in danger of losing our sense of self, our knowledge of our own vulnerability and limitations. If we entrust ourselves to the vast realm of nature, we realize how very small we are. As I had walked to Minamata City I had begun to see a part of myself that had been obscured by our fast-paced society. I learned that six hours of walking was all my body could take. In acknowledging how very small and fragile I am, I was able to restore the resonance that once existed between man and nature. My body welcomes the wind off the mountains. The smell of the tide fills my nostrils. My feet know the pain of hard use. I am comforted by the cries of birds overhead. I sense that my life is contained in the processes and cycles of the natural world.

Now that the so-called final settlement, the compromise position offered by the government, has been accepted by Minamata disease victims' groups, and now that the agreed-upon "onetime payment" has been distributed, the establishment eagerly awaits the day when the three characters representing "Minamata disease" are erased from public memory. At this time each victim of Minamata disease must confront the following question: "How will you continue to live your own Minamata disease in your own way?" For me, walking may provide one answer. Carving stone Buddhas is another way of expressing my own experience. It might be enough simply to place a stone, with reverence, on the reclaimed land. These actions are the words of my prayers, the gestures that define my vows, the means by which I etch my story in memory. We can plant trees, or add each day to a pile of small stones that, taken together, represent our collective experience. To be sure, in the eyes of those in the political world, these are actions of absolutely no significance. But they could not be more appropriate for those who have stopped entrusting their lives to our social establishment.

Until April, on the first day of each month I walked to the reclaimed land in Minamata City. After the third time, I stopped taking the dog and walked alone. The Japanese word for the first of the month, *tsuitachi*, contains the verb *tatsu*, "to depart, leave for," and so it had just the right sound for a day on which one would set out walking. May 1, 1996, was a special day, the fortieth anniversary of the "official discovery" of Minamata disease. Some time before this, however, my health had disintegrated.

When I finally regained my strength, I was ready for a new adventure. It was a crazy idea—navigating an *utasebune*—one of the traditional sailing vessels used for inshore fishing—through the outer waters all the way to Tokyo. *Uta-sabune*, a kind of trawler, are used for small-scale dragnet fishing. Hoisting four large sails, the crew relies on the power of the wind and the tides to drag small nets. The nets are designed to catch bottom-feeders like conger eel, squilla, and other shrimp. This fishing method dates back some four hundred years. The majority of *utasebune* are still made of wood. Of course, their numbers have dwindled since my childhood, but you can still find more than forty in my region. Today some of the boat owners have turned from fishing to tourism, using their boats for half-day excursions.

To mark the fortieth anniversary of Minamata disease, we all planned a great gathering, to be held that autumn, called the Minamata Tokyo Exposition. Many people who had been affiliated with the movement for some time were to play a central role, and preparations were under way. In February some of the organizers had come to tell me that they would like to exhibit an *utasebune* as one of the main attractions. It would be the best symbol for the exhibit, they said. They found someone who was willing to part with an old boat cheaply, but after looking into the matter, they learned that transporting the boat by truck or ship would be way beyond their budget.

What should they do? They didn't ask me up front, but I realized that they wanted to know if I would sail the boat to Tokyo. It was a crazy idea, but I asked them to give me two or three days to think about it. Of course, we all knew right from the start that I had inwardly accepted the offer. I saw it as a challenge. But no matter how I looked at it, the boat couldn't be sailed alone. I would need two or three other men, and they would have to be willing to entrust their lives to me.

I made my decision without even looking at the boat. I knew it was old, but I had been told that it had been fished until quite recently, so I figured it must be in fairly decent shape. A look at the boat proved otherwise. It would need a lot of repairs. To be honest, I was shocked.

Let me confess that I had never even been on one of these old fishing vessels. Because the *utasebune* is well known as the traditional fishing vessel of this region, outsiders think that all of the fishermen around here must still fish them. That's not the case. Even though we all fish the Shiranui Sea, each village has its traditional fishing methods. Some villages use seine nets, others gill nets, others drift nets, and others trawl nets. Moreover, this is all done by a permit system, so even if someone might like to introduce a new fishing method, it would be difficult. *Utase*-fishing is something that is passed down from father to son over generations. None of my clan, the Ogata fishermen, ever used *utasebune*. But because the craft were a part of my daily scenery, they felt familiar, and I didn't see why I couldn't learn to sail one.

I put out the word among *utase* fishermen that I needed a small crew to join me on a trip to Tokyo, but no one was willing. "No way," they said. Just the thought was terrifying. They couldn't believe I'd agreed to do this. *Utasebune* are designed only for inland seas. They float low in the water, and high waves and wind can capsize them. And, as I was to learn quite painfully later, their sails—designed to catch the crosswind so that the boat can drift while fishing—are absolutely useless for long-distance travel. Of course, the sails would be good for catching a tail wind, but then they would totally obstruct our view. I realized we would have to rely on an engine, but our boat came equipped with only a hundred-horsepower engine that could do eight knots—about as fast as pedaling slowly on a bicycle.

In the meantime, though, my plans were written up in the newspapers, and a father-and-son team from Miyazaki Prefecture offered to join me. The father was an experienced, licensed captain. Man, was I happy. After that, one of the young volunteers in the Minamata struggle and one of the office staff of the Minamata Tokyo Exposition volunteered. Including me, we now had a crew of five. It wasn't that we shared one vision. Each person had his own reasons for joining.

In my case, I had visited Okinawa, traveled to Europe, and walked from my home to the reclaimed land in Minamata. The Tokyo trip would be a continuation of those journeys. This time, however, I would board an unreliable ship and expose myself to the open sea, to the universe. This would be my way of participating in the Minamata Tokyo Exposition. In my heart I also felt like one of the sponsors. At a time when people thought of the Minamata incident as some past event, I wanted to confront society with questions that this incident had raised over the past forty years. What do we mean by "progress and civilization"? What is "modernization"? What does it mean to be human? I hoped that this unconventional—some might say, crazy—voyage on a traditional boat might provide a stimulus for rethinking these basic concepts. This boat, entrusted to such a mission, could not have borne a more suitable name. It had been christened *Nichigetsu-maru*, Boat of the Sun and the Moon.

I wanted to set sail in mid-July. Once you get into August, the probability of running into a typhoon increases. But the boat was in worse shape than I had imagined, and the repairs took time. It wouldn't do to rush things, so the day of our departure was set for August 6, the anniversary of the bombing of Hiroshima. Our route included stops at Nagasaki and Hiroshima, places we consciously linked with our consideration of the Minamata incident. As the day approached, our trip was featured in the papers, as well as on television and radio broadcasts. My friends stopped trying to dissuade me. Yet the pressure I felt continued to rise. Although I would leave the technical aspects of sailing to the captain, I was responsible for everything else. The fate of the crew was in my hands. At noon, one week before we were to sail, I looked up and saw rings around the sun. Others looked up and were equally surprised. This was the first time I had seen sun rings. They stood out clearly and beautifully. I took this as an omen and felt relieved.

At last, we set sail. We were prepared for the worst, but what happened next was totally unexpected. We had crossed the Shiranui Sea and were just about to head out to the ocean via the Hondo Strait when we hit an underwater barricade erected to block shifting sand. The propeller and its shaft were badly damaged. As we stood there in shock, the radio was still blaring something in the background about how the *Nichigetsu-maru* had made a stately departure that morning. Right! What were we going to do now? We used the boat's radio to search for an ironworks and finally located one, but due to the strong current going out through the strait, the boat hardly moved at all. We finally reached port, moving along at walking speed, and had the boat pulled out of the water. We were just feeling a bit better, thinking that we'd be off again soon, when the cable snapped just as the boat had been reeled to the top of the ramp. In an instant the *Nichigetsu-maru* slid right back into the sea.

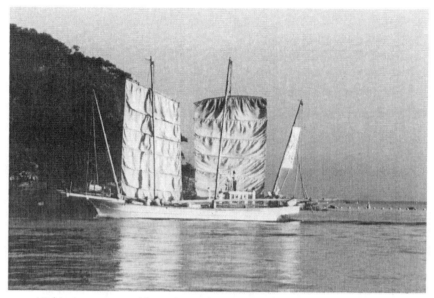

Nichigetsu-maru, an old utasebune, *departs Minamata Bay on August 6, 1996, for its arduous journey to Tokyo.*

Since most boats today are made of reinforced plastic, no one has facilities to handle heavy wooden boats. The folks at the ironworks were dreadfully embarrassed. And they were worried about trying it again. But somehow we persuaded them, and they agreed. They had heard about us on the news and sympathized with our situation. One of our crew, Kobayashi, was a diver, so he went under the boat and pulled up the cable. This time a second pulley was set up for extra power, and the boat came up safely. We exchanged the propeller shaft for a new one and were ready to go in three hours. We learned then that the accident had been a blessing in disguise. The old shaft had been badly corroded, and we might have found ourselves in worse trouble on the open sea. This incident made us understand our situation more clearly.

We headed north up the west coast of Kyushu, from Nagasaki to Sasebo, and then to Fukuoka. The weather wasn't bad, but about three times a day the whole crew had to work furiously to bail out the boat, even though we had repaired every leaky spot we could find. Once we passed through Kammon Strait into the Seto Inland Sea, we were in the milder seas for which this fishing boat was designed, and our work became easier. On the other hand, the large sails proved a liability when we tried to pass between islands or other fishing vessels. A sailboat has to set its course by the wind, so it can be difficult to navigate in narrow channels. We cooked and slept on board.

If it rained hard at night, we would all be soaked by morning. We all cursed this boat, which had one problem after another, and I'm sure there were times when the crew regretted their decisions to join me. Still, we had no arguments, and we managed to hold together until the end.

The real test came when we hit the rough waters of the Pacific. What had come before now seemed like a luxury cruise. I had never seen such swells! Waves piled on waves. Even nearby boats were lost from sight in the deep troughs. The four masts swayed violently as the boat was tossed on the waves, and they began to come loose at their bases. We would scramble to fix them as we went along, and it seems like a miracle now that we didn't lose any. There wasn't a moment when we weren't bailing water or repairing something. When we finally found ourselves face to face with a typhoon, we managed to escape into a fishing port to wait out the bad weather.

There were good times, too. We caught lots of fish, so we were never short of food. When we pulled into ports for the night, local fishermen would gather around, curious about our unusual boat. They would offer us good things to eat and drink. To them, our vessel must have seemed like something from the dinosaur age. A wooden boat with sails has become a rarity all over Japan, and ours, in tatters and shreds, must have presented quite a spectacle. To make it even stranger, we were flying a large banner. "The Sea and the Human Mind Must Regenerate," it said. People who read the message offered their encouragement.

There were some people, though, who held us in suspicion. We were always on the radio announcing who we were and what we were doing. Toward the end of our journey, just off Ito, we couldn't make headway through the high waves. A maritime patrol boat approached, and right before their eyes a rotten board in the side of our boat popped out, jarred loose by the rocking waves. They radioed to ask where we'd come from and told us they were towing us in for inspection. They did, and when we arrived we showed them our papers, the captain's license, and the news clippings about our trip, but they were not convinced and insisted on looking around the boat. They must have thought we were carrying refugees. We used the inspection to our advantage and made some needed repairs. It turned out that we were in a resort marina, with nothing but luxury boats. In this company the *Nichigetsu-maru* looked pathetic even to our eyes.

Thirteen days and 1,500 kilometers later, we arrived in Tokyo, where we promptly collapsed from fatigue and relief. Shortly afterward I returned to Kumamoto, as it would still be a month before the exposition opened. Someone had to stay and bail out the boat, though, or it would have sunk. The younger crewmen checked on the boat every day.

The evening before the opening of the Minamata Tokyo Exposition, a ceremony was held to welcome the spirits of those who had died from organic mercury poisoning. This lively ceremony took place under a full moon. An easterly breeze blew through the valleys of Tokyo's tall buildings, filling the sails of the *Nichigetsu-maru,* which had been raised onto land for the exposition. Candles lit up paper lanterns, and a Noh drum reverberated through the night.

Together with Tsuchimoto Noriaki's photographs of five hundred deceased Minamata disease victims, the *Nichigetsu-maru* was the focal point of the Minamata Tokyo Exposition. I wanted this exposition to serve as a point of release or liberation from the anguish of the past. We owed this to the spirits of deceased villagers who had accompanied us on our boat. Shinagawa, our exposition site, was land reclaimed from the sea, a fate it shared with a large portion of Minamata Bay. Nearby was a huge crane, and all around were tall buildings. Below these stood our wooden boat with its battered sails. The juxtaposition alone carried a strong message.

At the end of the exposition the *Nichigetsu-maru,* which had played its final role, was torn apart on-site and hauled off to an incinerator. There we held a kind of funeral, to see off the spirits it had borne to Tokyo. I would like to have sunk it in the sea, so that it might have served as a nursery for fish, but we could not get permission. I am still amazed that our boat survived the open seas. I think the most important reason was the significance of its mission. It had been my responsibility to fulfill the villagers' wish that I convey the spirits of their deceased to the exposition. These villagers had gathered at the reclaimed land to see us off. One of my relatives called out, "Are you spirits all aboard? This is a special voyage—you mustn't miss the boat!"

As we sailed we had always been conscious of having spirits among us. Although one of our crew may have stood at the wheel, it was the spirits who moved the boat along. They were not only the spirits of humans but also of fish, birds, and cats—all the creatures poisoned by organic mercury.

Many people have questioned my motives for this voyage, even my family. I have a hard time explaining it myself. Rumors had spread that I was paid a lot of money; but if money had been involved, I would have refused from the outset. The voyage itself didn't really sink in until some time later. Thinking back on it now always cheers me up. It was dangerous but worth every minute. Look how far our civilized society has come in its search for comfort and safety. We can't shirk a little danger if we are to oppose contemporary values.

The Chisso within Us

Japan is a society that likes to settle its accounts with the past. In the case of the Minamata incident, the government sought closure through the final settlement reached in 1995. But, I strongly believe that there can never be a final act in the tragedy of Minamata. In order to explain my position, I will review the history of Minamata disease, relating certain patterns to my interpretation of current circumstances.

The history of Minamata disease can be divided roughly into three periods. During the initial period, from the late 1950s to around 1973, the victims had no other recourse than to fight directly with Chisso. First of all, the fishermen demanded that Chisso stop releasing untreated effluent. In November 1959 the patients themselves staged a sit-in demonstration in front of the main gate to the factory. At the end of December, they concluded the "sympathy contract" with Chisso. After this there was a period of silence. Then, in 1968, the government established a pollution-certification process, which became the springboard for patients to take on Chisso in court. The first lawsuit was filed concerning the outbreak of Minamata disease in Kumamoto Prefecture. In 1973 the case was decided in favor of the plaintiffs. In parallel with these events, sit-ins were staged in 1971 at the Minamata Chisso factory and at the main office in Tokyo by people who advocated independent negotiations with Chisso. These collective efforts resulted in the compensation agreement of July 1973, which stipulated a onetime payment of sixteen to eighteen million yen per certified victim, depending on the severity of symptoms. The agreement included a clause stating that patients certified in the future would be entitled to the same amount. Chisso fought this clause but in the end was forced to accept it. The patients who fought hard in this first stage of the incident left the reparation system as their legacy.

The second stage begins in 1974, when Chisso devised an elaborate certification system for individuals seeking compensation. During this period the patients' struggle focused on the certification procedure, and their primary

143

opponent was Kumamoto Prefecture. Time and again they brought into question the fairness of decisions handed down by a government-appointed certification board, the long delays in the certification process, and the extent to which the government bore responsibility for the incident. As soon as the Minamata Disease Certification Applicants' Council was formed in 1974, I became a member and played a leading role in the struggle. We argued over standards for certification. Chisso and the prefectural government called for very strict criteria, while the patients and their support groups asked for recognition of actual harm done to the individual. Until this time the national government had never shown its face.

The third stage dates from 1978, when Chisso found itself unable to make reparation payments. Heavily in debt, Chisso appealed to the prefectural and national governments, whereupon the prefecture began floating loans to the company. From that time on Chisso ceased to be an independent company and proceeded to absorb eighteen billion yen in relief funds. What was new at this stage was the appearance of the national government. It was strange, indeed, that the state had not taken a position on this incident earlier, but now it was drawn into the arena by the prefecture, with demands for financial assistance and an independent certification council at the national level. Twice the Kumamoto Prefectural Assembly refused to conduct certification. At last the state created a separate certification council within the Environment Agency. Ultimately, then, the patients had to deal with three different faces: Chisso, the prefecture, and the national government.

In 1980, after struggling with the compensation system and pleading with the state to accept responsibility, over two thousand patients became plaintiffs in a huge lawsuit demanding compensation from the national government, the prefecture, and Chisso. What had heretofore been direct negotiations shifted to the courtroom.

Although the Kumamoto court ruled in favor of the plaintiffs in 1987 and the responsibilities of the state and prefecture were recognized, the government immediately appealed the case. There were many who felt they could not endure the prolonged legal process, and this group decided not to litigate further but to take a "path of reconciliation" toward a political settlement. This led to the state's final-settlement plan reached in 1995, concluding negotiations between Chisso and the patients.

As we look back on these events, we see that Minamata disease became something that could not be discussed except in the courtroom or within the certification process. In both venues, the bottom line was money. Isn't this the case throughout Japanese society today, even in other environmental movements?

As the struggle evolved from the first to the third stage, Chisso itself evolved from a private enterprise to a kind of quasi-public operation propped up by prefectural bonds. The bonds could not be redeemed for five years but would reach maturity in thirty years. To repay the original bonds, the prefecture would issue another set of bonds. Supported by this ongoing cycle of loans, Chisso became something like a phoenix, whose life is renewed each time it dies. The company never had any intention of paying back the loans received to compensate the victims and clean up the environment. In order to fulfill the requirements of the 1995 final settlement, the government is still supporting Chisso. This is the same way it bails out savings and loan institutions and banks. Chisso became a microcosm of the system—a system in which Minamata disease had become fully entrenched.

From the time I applied for certification in 1974 until I withdrew my application in 1986, I played an active role in this history. I had to withdraw so that I too would not be engulfed by this system. In our movement we were fighting to determine responsibility for Minamata disease. But it gradually became clear to me that Chisso, the prefecture, and the national government could respond only from within the system, that it was impossible for any of them to accept fundamental responsibility. Since we could not pinpoint the locus of responsibility, we began to focus on financial compensation. The compensation system was designed to substitute and cover up for those who should have accepted responsibility. I could no longer bear to be a part of it.

The idea of assuming responsibility is an illusion. Our legal proceedings are premised on this illusion. We make the assumption that if we pay reparations, we have assumed responsibility. But, if not money, what? I believe that until recently to accept responsibility meant to share the pain one caused another. But today, in order to avoid the pain, we turn the situation into a business negotiation. "Just take this money and put up with your lot," we say, dismissing the sufferers from our thoughts. Responsibility is exchanged for money, and something crucial is lost in the process. I withdrew my application to deny the validity of this exchange.

Let me add, however, that I have no intention of denying the significance of our search for responsibility through the movement. This was very important as an expression of our anger as victims. And applicants who continued to fight for their rights did make headway. For example, they were granted medical expenses while they waited for certification. Still, these achievements belong to a different dimension than that of establishing ultimate responsibility.

When we speak of the state's responsibility or of Chisso's responsibility, we have to consider the questions of who, when, and where. Can we definitively say when Minamata disease began? Was it in 1908, when the first Chisso factory was built in Minamata? Was it in 1932, when Chisso first began using methyl mercury as a catalyst? When we, in the movement, speak of the responsibility of Chisso, or the national government, or prefecture, or city, we are referring to a kind of organizational responsibility. Yet at the bottom of this organization ultimately there must be human accountability. It is not the responsibility of a particular person in a particular time and place but a deeper, more abstract responsibility borne by the human race.

I'm not questioning the government's responsibility to pay compensation. But even if it is judged that the government is responsible, it will never be clear who this government is. It is impossible to clarify the locus of responsibility. To pursue responsibility is like pursuing an apparition that constantly changes its shape. In this endless pursuit you can lose your own soul. Rather than chase ghosts, it is better to stand firm and declare, "I am a human being! I am a mirror of who you are."

Generally we see sin or guilt as something to be avoided. I look upon sin in a more positive way. It is something we all bear and will carry with us as long as we live. We need to face this sin and live with it, just as we need to face the fact that our demands for the assumption of responsibility are meaningless. I too pressed Chisso and the state to admit their responsibility. But now I ask myself the question, "If I had worked for Chisso or within the government administration, is it possible that I would have behaved exactly as they did?" I cannot deny the possibility. Doesn't this mean that I carry Chisso within me? I am forced to conclude that human beings bear the sin for Minamata disease and that the fundamental responsibility for this incident lies in the nature of our collective existence. When human beings no longer look upon one another as fellow humans, then we each become responsible for such incidents as Minamata disease. When we are part of a movement, we forget to look into ourselves. From the perspective of the movement, Chisso is the Other, the enemy, the assailant. For me, this viewpoint evolved until I could recognize "the Chisso within."

What is all the commotion we've been hearing about the final settlement of 1995? Let's take a closer look. This "final settlement" refers to a political compromise designed to provide relief to patients of Minamata disease who had not yet been recognized by the prefecture or state. In the summer of 1995, a coalition of political parties presented a compromise agreement to the various victims' groups and to Chisso. By autumn, the five principal groups had agreed to the terms of the compromise.

Politicians looked upon this as "a speedy and total solution to the Minamata disease struggle." These were essentially the same words used by victims' and supporters' groups when they lodged their "mammoth lawsuit for state indemnities." The mass media grabbed these phrases and proceeded to shape public opinion. The city, towns, and villages all decided to go for a compromise settlement. Just about every regional group joined the chorus—labor unions, chambers of commerce, women's organizations. "Reach a final settlement through compromise. Keep Chisso alive. Revitalize the region." Most of the victims' groups went along. From schools to the workplace—any place was fair ground for consciousness raising. It was made to appear that public opinion was moving the government, but in reality the government was shaping public opinion. A speedy conclusion to the Minamata incident was exactly what the government wanted. I wondered if this wasn't exactly how the fascist regime of wartime Japan manipulated public opinion.

The central points of the final settlement were that ten thousand noncertified patients would agree to a onetime payment of 2.6 million yen each and that the municipalities of Minamata and Ashikita would together receive 30 billion yen. This money was to come from national and prefectural taxes. The money for the patients, however, was not to be distributed to them directly. A foundation to be established in Kumamoto Prefecture would loan the money to Chisso, and the company was to pay the patients. The company was to repay the loans over fifty years.

Until this point the patients had sought admissions from Chisso, the prefecture, and the national government that they were all responsible for this pollution incident. This demand was expressed in one court after another. If we look at the history of Minamata disease, it is quite clear that the corporation, the prefecture, and the state are all perpetrators of this crime, but of the six court verdicts passed so far, the national government is cited for negligence in only three. In the final settlement, the state avoided facing up to its responsibility, and the patients gave up their right to pursue the issue farther in the courts.

Were those sufferers who had pursued the certification process for years now considered legitimate patients? Certainly not. Even today they are not recognized as Minamata disease patients. On the other hand, their status cannot be denied. The government referred to them as "patients receiving relief as a result of the settlement." The media referred to "the issue of relief for patients not officially certified." The money paid out was therefore a kind of relief, in the form of a onetime payment. This is a nebulous world, where there is neither assault nor injury.

All of this reflects the power of money. At the same time, we also see a reflection of our times. As social pressure rose to bring the Minamata incident to a close, the patients themselves reached the limits of fatigue. I understand the feelings of those who had grown old, and of those who were weary of the long years of struggle. What would happen if they were to reject this compromise solution? They could not read the future. Public opinion favored a settlement, and to stand in opposition would be to break step with one's group. If one stood up as an individual, one would become totally isolated. Patients may have been attracted to the money, but their fear of being ostracized was even stronger.

The state, prefecture, and Chisso didn't even have to convince the patients. They left that to the respective victims' groups. It just took a little political pressure on top of existing social pressure to get the various local groups to control their members. In other words, the Minamata disease movement was now totally controlled within a framework created by Chisso, the prefecture, and the state. It wasn't exactly a reward, but in addition to the 2.6 million yen allotted to each patient, the five main victims' groups each received a considerable sum of money, in proportion to membership.

More people than I would ever have imagined surged forward to fill out "applications for relief" in accordance with the terms of the final settlement. There must have been more than thirteen thousand. My village was no different. Everyone was out to get something. It was as if they were all going out to buy lottery tickets, after which they would compare their luck. No one had any compunction about applying—after all, everyone was doing it. Earlier on, one of my older sisters had decided that she would not apply. She believed in my position. But people tend to move together. She felt left behind. She changed her mind, "because my other brothers and sisters convinced me that this was best." "That's fine," I told her. "I'm not going to find fault with you. You don't need to think you've let me down. It's your decision. It's just that I have to follow my own path."

Then, after some time, my wife's brothers and sisters started working on her, saying, "Why don't you apply? You're going to miss the boat." "If you don't apply now, there won't be another chance," they warned. Sawako consulted me about all this, and I told her not to apply. "If you do, I'll divorce you." Sawako agreed, and I felt relieved. About half a year passed, and at some point she did apply—secretly, of course. She qualified for the onetime payment, and when the notice arrived, she thought she'd better confess. She approached me fearfully and told me what she'd done. I blew up. But, after yelling until I was red in the face, I said no more. Even in the case of husband and wife, the final decision has to be up to the individual.

There were people who encouraged me to apply, out of what appeared to be the kindest of motives. I would just laugh. There were probably some who thought I really should undergo a change of heart and accept the money. I understood what they were up to. If I had applied for the money, there wouldn't be a single person left to say, "The Minamata disease incident is not yet over."

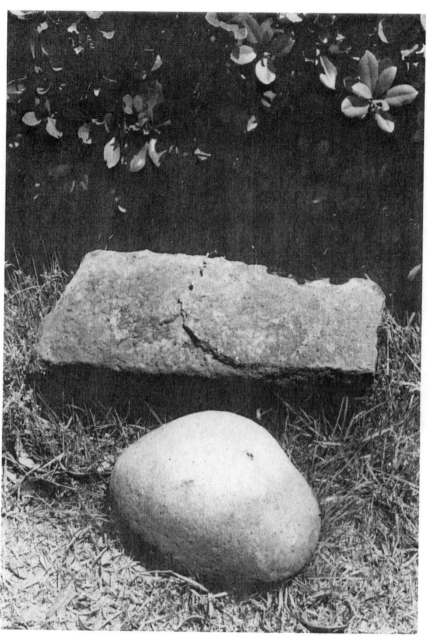

Rocks placed in prayer on the reclaimed land by a Minamata-disease victim

I wouldn't be truthful if I didn't own up to thinking that all those people who rushed to apply for reparations were utterly lacking in self-respect. But I can't very well blame them. I think that the movement that had led the patients to this point bears a lot of the responsibility. That the movement was guilty of labeling these fishing people as "certified patients," or "patients who have applied for certification," or "plaintiffs," and pulling them into the system cannot be denied. However, my anger is really directed at the state and its authority, for pressing my friends and family and neighbors into a corner. The authorities dragged the trials and negotiations on and on, exhausting the patients both physically and financially, and then offered onetime payments to silence them forever. Patients were divided up and ranked according to diagnoses and their affiliations with particular groups, and pressure was applied from within each organization. With what skill and callousness the authorities executed their high-handed tactics! This is what infuriates me. It's as if the government had herded our souls onto a reservation.

When I think about it, though, I realize that this situation is not limited to Minamata disease. All movements must share these problems. In labor movements people are reduced to "laborers," and in women's movements people are categorized as "women." I'm not denying the value of these movements. Each movement has played a particular role in social history. On the other hand, each movement is limited to a given social context. There isn't any movement that goes on forever. Before we are Minamata disease patients, we are laborers. Before that we are women. Before that we are human beings. And as human beings, we are but single components of the greater web of Life.

Keep the Embers Glowing

It was about ten days before his death that I learned that my friend Kawamoto Teruo had been hospitalized. I heard that his cancer had progressed and his time was running out. The doctors could do no more than administer sedatives to kill the pain, and his consciousness was growing dim. I don't recall him ever mentioning that he felt bad. He died on February 18, 1999. I was not alone in thinking that death had taken him far too suddenly.

I must have been twenty when I first met Kawamoto. I was at the height of youth, reckless and bold. As I mentioned earlier, his presence greatly influenced my decision to get involved in the Minamata struggle. For nearly twelve years I fought at Kawamoto's side. Almost everyone has vivid memories of him as a leader of the Minamata movement. Of course, I also remember him in this role, but for me there are special, personal memories as well. There was quite an age difference between us, but we shared special moments together that I will treasure always. It was Kawamoto who tempered my character.

When I withdrew my application for certification in 1985, I went to Kawamoto to tell him my decision. I hoped that although I would be leaving the movement, our paths would cross again. I continued to harbor this hope, but he passed on before my wish could be realized. I will always regret that we never got to face each other again and work things out.

I had heard that in the years before Kawamoto's death a number of acquaintances had parted ways with him, leaving him with a sense of isolation. I could understand his anguish. I heard through one of my nephews, who lived near Kawamoto and was quite close to him, that Kawamoto had been saying he'd like to get together with me. I let my nephew know that I'd like to join him for a drink. My nephew carried the messages back and forth, but the timing never seemed right. I thought that if Kawamoto decided not to run for city council in the April election, this would create a good opportunity for us to get together. He had already served three terms, and I heard that he was debating whether to run a fourth time. If he didn't run we would be able to meet as two ordinary citizens and speak our minds freely. That was my hope.

The funeral was held at Kawamoto's home. The house was overflowing. I heard later that more than a thousand people came to mourn his passing. Many were crying. I understood how they felt, but I could not cry. There were so many topics we had left unaddressed. I felt only emptiness. It wasn't until some time after the funeral that the tears finally came.

The house was so crowded during the wake and the funeral that there was no opportunity to speak with Kawamoto's family. Later I learned from my nephew that Kawamoto's wife and son wanted me to have some of Kawamoto's personal belongings as mementos. I returned to their house. Aside from chance encounters on the street, this was the first time in thirteen years that I had met Mrs. Kawamoto. The day I visited happened to be the Seventh Day memorial service, and the priest had just left. Incense lingered in the air. After taking off my shoes, I asked permission to offer incense and pray at the family altar. Mrs. Kawamoto told me that her husband had been very run down and that his drinking had increased considerably over the past two or three years. "You'll ruin your health if you keep drinking like that," she had warned him, but he couldn't stop. Listening to her talk, I could feel his pain and loneliness. I left with Kawamoto's favorite Panama hat and necktie.

I imagine that in those last few years the Minamata issue must have brought considerable anguish to the Kawamoto household. Even within the movement, Kawamoto had been increasingly misunderstood and isolated. During those years Minamata was chanting the mantra of compromise. Everyone—from laborers to lawyers, from government administrators to Parent–Teacher Association mothers, and even the patients themselves—was waving three banners, calling for "a rapid, final settlement," "economic stability for Chisso," and "regional revitalization." These voices grew so loud that it became increasingly difficult to express a different opinion. Engulfed by this fervor, the patients and their supporters must have found Kawamoto's presence disagreeable—after all, it was he who had led the litigation struggle for so many years when the patients had sought not only financial relief but admission of responsibility. In this atmosphere Kawamoto found himself in a situation in which he could neither clearly approve nor disapprove of the compromise settlement. As a member of the Minamata city council, he had one foot in government administration. He was also a member of the council's Special Committee for Pollution Countermeasures. I imagine he must have questioned all the effort he had devoted to the movement for so many years.

There is no doubt, however, that Kawamoto admirably fulfilled his leadership role in the Minamata movement, a role for which he had been cast by a set of unusual circumstances, and that he played to his greatest possible credit. By exposing the prejudice and discrimination experienced by the victims as well as their own struggles for self-esteem, Kawamoto forced the company, the government, and society to recognize the human face of Minamata disease, and he was in large part responsible for securing its place on Japan's political map.

When the final settlement plan was formulated, it gave the impression that the Minamata incident was over. In this context, the death of someone who had played such a pivotal role in the struggle seemed to mark a turning point. Now we must ask ourselves: What are the burdens we continue to bear? What meaning can we extract from our long years of struggle, and how can we each go on living with our own Minamata disease? Kawamoto's Panama hat hangs on a wall in my study. I feel it looking down on me, urging me to be strong.

As I look back on the Minamata movement, or at current nuclear-power and dam-construction issues, I always wonder why people give in to money. Why do they settle for compensation funds or "onetime" settlement payments? What does *hosho*, compensation, mean? I have been thinking about this for a long time. I think "compensation" is a concept that entered Japan in the Meiji period, along with other concepts of modernization and Westernization. Earlier, under the oppressive authority structure of feudal Japan, one had no choice but to accept one's lot—or die. It would be a mistake, however, to think that the compensation system had been forced on the people from above. It was one of the citizens' demands in the process of democratization, and it is something we continue to demand today. We have sought out a lifestyle in which everything has a price.

Today almost all workers have been swallowed up by the Establishment, and you seldom hear anyone speak of "class struggle." You can no longer distinguish the political Right from the Left. As the economy grows, demands for compensation will increase both in number and amount. However, as capital plays a greater role in our lives, the place occupied by the soul seems to shrink. This is a situation that we, the people, have created in collaboration with the Establishment.

Of course, the reason we seek compensation is that we feel we cannot get by without it. Perhaps it has become a rite of passage, concluding an event. When a person dies, we hold a wake and a funeral, followed by seventh-day, forty-ninth-day, and one-year Buddhist memorial services. Perhaps compensation is also a ritual. In this sense it does have meaning.

I've given a lot of thought to those who received compensation and one-time payments. In one group you find those who sought compensation not simply to make a profit but because they considered it a fine or penalty for Chisso's actions. Similarly, there were those who sought compensation through the certification process. The second group followed the first, mainly for the sake of the money itself. In other words, while the first group pressed for admission of responsibility and settled for compensation, withdrawing into their own hearts without receiving the compassion they sought, the second group accepted money without concerning themselves with responsibility. The question still remains, however, as to why no one went one step farther, why no one kicked in the wall of the system, exclaiming, "This isn't about money!" There are some who received payment and then said, "This isn't about money." But how can you extract yourself from the system once you have been paid off?

I feel that I understand these people better today. It is said that ours is only one of an infinite number of worlds contained within the palm of the Buddha. The Buddha hides this from us out of compassion, knowing how much we would suffer if we had to face the whole truth. We think our world and our own lives are of utmost importance. But from the perspective of infinite time and space, our position is totally insignificant. Probably those who received compensation, especially those who had been in the vanguard of the movement, sensed that as long as they held to the line that they were not after money, they would be exposing themselves to extreme suffering. They must have realized what would lie ahead: expulsion from society, isolation, and ultimately insanity. I understand this only too well from my own experience. Because they could foresee this fate, they chose to accept the money and withdraw their feelings into the inner recesses of their hearts. Who am I to censure their actions?

I feel the same way about those who continued in the movement after I left. By the time they pursued a compromise settlement, the situation had become far more complex than it had been when we were struggling with Chisso over responsibility. Toward the end, the movement had lost almost all of its supporters. and the mass media was calling loudly for a rapid, compromise settlement. In these circumstances it would have been very difficult to maintain that you were holding out for something more than money.

Therefore, rather than seeing the victims "taking money," I see them as "withdrawing." After waiting patiently for years in the most difficult conditions and enduring all the accusations surrounding their motives, they found themselves accepting a final settlement. Their own feelings were in turmoil, and the Minamata incident itself was left unresolved. Each person's share amounted to no more than 2.6 million yen. It was not a question of money. Having no one to entrust themselves to, the patients withdrew into themselves. They didn't flee. They returned home.

There is no need for us to be obsessed with the words "Minamata disease" for the rest of our lives. Just as we must free ourselves from the system, so we must free ourselves of Minamata disease. We need to let go and return to the lives of ordinary people. If I think about those who accepted the final payment in this way, it all makes sense.

There is no way I can be indifferent toward my friends who struggled until the bitter end for certification. There's no need for anyone to feel guilty about receiving a sum of money that would barely purchase a car. They should think of the money as "travel expenses." That's about all that will be left after they pay their legal fees. How could anyone blame them for accepting a settlement after they had been kept waiting for twenty to thirty years?

People of greatly varying characters live in a multitude of different circumstances. So I want to call out to everyone in the Minamata movement, "It's all right. Just come on home!" You don't have to come home with some kind of diploma. When sons go to war, mothers say, "Don't worry about what you achieve. Just come home." Even if they return empty-handed, their mothers rejoice. It doesn't matter what they did, as long as they return safely. This is the big-hearted welcome I would like to give those returning from the movement. But unlike that period marking the end of the Pacific War, we can't welcome home our soldiers with the words, "While you were gone the fish have increased!" It is quite the opposite today. If there were more fish, even those who had left for the cities would return.

In the past when I used expressions like "the Chisso within us" and "the state is but another expression for ourselves," people challenged me with the question, "Does that mean, then, that you have forgiven your enemies?" Naturally, it's not easy to forgive one's enemies. For those whose very existences are determined in relation to their enemies, to lose their enemies would be to lose their own identities. That's a terrifying prospect. When I applied for certification I was not yet aware of this. I was still young.

But I did not forgive the authorities. I simply threw them out of my life. I don't find the state valuable enough to want to keep on pursuing it. The state makes no attempt to assume responsibility and, in fact, is incapable of doing so. It gives you some kind of glib response, but that's not what the patients want to hear. What they want is compassion—someone to share their pain. There is an unbridgeable gap between the individual and the system. You must place your trust in one side or the other. I place my trust in the individual.

When I withdrew my application for certification, there were those who criticized me, saying, "All you are doing is satisfying the state and the company." I certainly don't see it that way. I acted to divorce myself from the state. There are still people who, as long as they live, will never say, "It's over." These people cannot be judged by the standards of the Establishment. The system is at a loss as to how to deal with them. They don't put their trust in the state but in themselves. This is also a form of resistance.

The Japanese system has become so stifling that it's no wonder people want radical social change. But whenever I think of embarking on this course, I find myself short of breath. I remember what happened to me when I was in the movement—I was always making plans, trying to influence someone. What I have learned is to pay attention to today, to make the best of each moment. Every evening I give thanks for surviving one more day. It's best not to try to control the future.

But to live each moment fully is to live in a way that will benefit future generations. The future is built on today. This is part of the wisdom of traditional peoples. They knew that the cedar seedling they transplanted today would be used one or two hundred years later. They behaved this way naturally, without conscious thought or effort.

When my father was still well he would rub his forehead on my own, softly chanting, "pass on, pass on." He was transmitting a bit of his soul to me. He must have thought that it would give me strength when I needed it. I believe it is because I spent six years in this way with my father that I have had the strength to survive some pretty hard times. People today may think this transmission of souls is strange, but in the past it was a common ritual. Many indigenous peoples believe they have been able to survive precisely because their ancestors transferred their souls from generation to generation. Even during times of persecution they continued to transmit their souls, and that spiritual light remains undimmed today.

Although traditional peoples may lament the death of loved ones, they believe that they will always be connected to their ancestors through their common soul. They believe that all things, including their own lives and deaths, are indivisibly linked. When we talk about "teaching" or "transmitting," we refer to actions performed at a conscious level. We refer to the communication of knowledge. But the real question is, how do we transmit a deeper level of understanding?

Society whispers in our ear, "It's all over. Forget it." The Minamata disease incident is only one example. Society loves to find some sense of closure for all these issues and to seal them away forever. But we can't let it happen. We'll puncture their seal—even a small hole in a can will cause the contents to rot. It is this very kind of resistance that makes spiritual transmission possible.

Traditional peoples have been cast aside and marginalized the world over. Their numbers may be few, but their existence has become ever more meaningful. Those who remain are like embers. They are the coals that we save to light the next fire. They may be in the minority, but in the last analysis everyone has to stand alone. When the system tells me, "It's all over. The fire is out," I want to be right here to declare, "No. Here are the embers. I've kept them glowing."

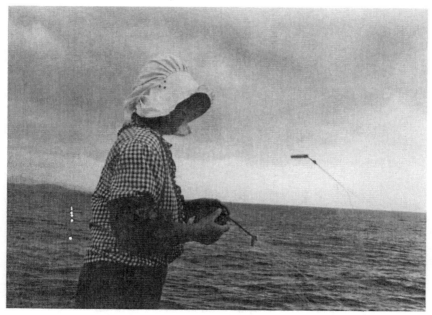

Masato's wife, Sawako, casts a net in the Shiranui Sea.

Nusari, Embracing Life as a Gift

A number of years ago a film crew from NHK television came to visit my mother at Meisuien, a live-in nursing facility for certified Minamata disease patients. Mother must have heard that I had been to Tokyo recently, because she turned to me and said, "I didn't know you could fish in Tokyo!"

Her words took me by surprise, and I was so embarrassed that I didn't know quite how to reply. Fumbling for words, I said, "Why would there be any fish in a place like that?" Deep inside, I was shaken. Her words revealed that Tokyo meant nothing to her; it was as meaningless as a fart. She had simply concluded that if her son had gone there, it must have fish. Most people consider Tokyo with awe. It's the political center of Japan. Her words expressed harsh criticism against contemporary Japanese, myself included.

My mother used to say, "Don't worry about other people's business. Just swat the flies from your own face." This was her philosophy. For example, when candidates or their backers would canvass the neighborhoods before elections, Mother would say, "Elections these days are really annoying. In the old days these things had nothing to do with us women, so why bother us now?" Another question she liked to repeat when I was involved in the movement was, "If you can catch fish, grow sweet potatoes, and eat your fill, isn't that enough?"

These words didn't really sink in until I suffered a nervous breakdown in 1985. Until then I had just thought of my mother as a country bumpkin, the very picture of narrow-mindedness and ignorance. After all, she had left our region only twice in her life. The first time was at age eighteen or nineteen, when she went to visit her sister in Kyoto. The other was when she came to see me in jail, after my arrest in Kumamoto. She was always busy—in the fields, with the fish, in the house. Her life left no time to think. Even when she complained, it never occurred to her that there was anything wrong with society. On the contrary, I gave a lot of thought to social injustice. In the end, though, we arrived at the same conclusion. Strange, isn't it?

Speaking of small worlds—victims of congenital Minamata disease live

159

very constricted lives. Take my nephew, Tatsuzumi. He spent about three months in Meisuien when he was a child, but other than that he has spent his entire life at home. Of course, this is a huge burden on his family. He lives in Kyodomari, around the point from my house. His mother (my sister) and her husband have a house on the shore, and Tatsuzumi lives in a small annex in the back. Aside from cooking he's able to look after himself. His mother brings his meals. He's become so heavy that it's difficult for one person to help him move around, and he doesn't get much opportunity to go outside. Besides, he tires easily and gets both seasick and carsick, so he's reluctant to travel anywhere. Sunning himself on the verandah is his limit.

Tatsuzumi's feet are curved inward, making it impossible for him to stand. His hands are curled up as well, but somehow he is able to support himself with his stronger arm and sit up. He's never been to school, although a teacher who is a friend of the family did come to tutor him in basic education for many years. Writing is impossible, and he can barely read. He understands what people say to him, but his speaking ability is limited. His ability to read people's hearts, though, is extraordinary.

Tatsuzumi's strength is in his eyes. Sometimes his face takes on the appearance of a Noh mask, and his eyes seem to pierce right through you. Although

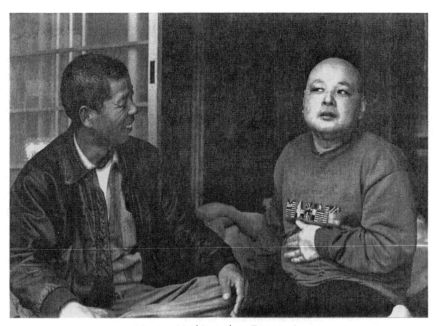

Masato visits his nephew Tatsuzumi.

he isn't like this all the time, it can be rather unnerving. It's as if he possesses a power of expression that transcends language; his eyes seem to expose my overreliance on the spoken word.

I think that Tatsuzumi and I have a special connection. We're almost the same age, so rather than uncle and nephew, we're more like brothers. He even calls me "An-chan," older brother. From the time I was a child, I saw the hardships Tatsuzumi's parents endured to care for him. I began to hate Chisso. I swore to take revenge on those who had killed my father and made Tatsuzumi and his family suffer. Tatsuzumi's grandparents adored him, and it was probably because they wanted so much to help him that they were both very long-lived. They worried about him until they died. "Masato," they would say, "We're counting on you. Take care of Tatsuzumi after we're gone." When Tatsuzumi's grandmother died, I was asked to read her will. In it she said, "I die with great concern for Tatsuzumi, and I will continue to worry about him in the next life and worlds to come."

Partly because of the trust shown me by his parents and grandparents, Tatsuzumi has always had complete faith in me. He knows that I've been active in the Minamata movement. Perhaps he thinks I'm doing his share too. He trusts me to speak for him, not hiding anything. Nowadays I don't visit Tatsuzumi very often. But when I was "going mad" in 1985, I stopped by frequently. Although I wasn't conscious of it, I think I was hoping that Tatsuzumi would share some special kind of understanding with me. At that time it was only Tatsuzumi who saw that I was close to death. "An-chan is in danger," he told my older sister. "He might die."

Tatsuzumi keeps a pretty tight daily schedule. He seems to resist any socially imposed schedule but rather invents one to suit his taste. Tatsuzumi has infinite patience. He has the power to wait until someone at last understands him. In this information age, we become increasingly impatient—we want more news, faster than before. Our ability to wait, to be patient, has weakened. In Japanese the verb "to wait" and the noun "pine tree" are both pronounced *matsu*. Look how strong pines are, growing on rocky, wind-swept cliffs. Even when sprayed by salty waves, they endure.

That's why I believe that although Tatsuzumi's world is narrow, it is deep. There's a saying, "The frog in the well does not know the sea." The second part goes: "But it knows the depths of the well." Tatsuzumi may be short on words, but his existence itself speaks to me. When we break through that framework we call society and the state and discover who we are and in what we can trust—this is where we will find Tatsuzumi.

It is the same in the case of my mother. The purity with which these two humans live their lives, against the natural backdrop of their native village,

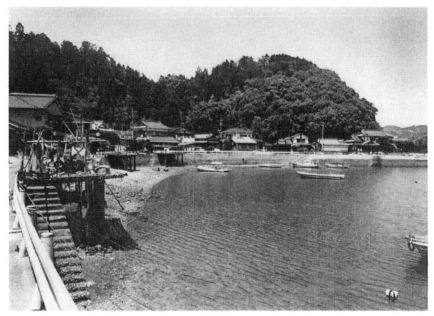

The hamlet of Kyodomari, where Masato's relatives, including his nephew Tatsuzumi, live

sends me the message that we can cut ourselves free. We can live without the state, fully interacting with the fields, the mountains, and the sea.

In recent years a mountain of discussion and research has grown around Minamata disease. Even today people ask, "So, what is the lesson of Minamata disease?" Or, "How would you sum up the Minamata movement?" After all this time, I'm not sure that such discussions have any value. To begin with, I hate moralizing. Moreover, I feel that this incident crushed us beyond the point that it was possible to moralize. According to whose or what criteria would the incident be judged? We are not interested in any more bogus standards of measurement. Such criteria would measure only the shallowness of human wisdom.

As I look back, however, I do see three distinct characteristics of the Minamata disease incident. If we were to "sum it up," I believe these three features would suffice. First of all, when news got out about "a strange disease" and consumers stopped buying fish, the people of our fishing villages continued to eat the fish. Second, when a first child and then a second was born with Minamata disease, we gave birth to a third and then a fourth child, raising them all with love and care. Each was a *takarago*, a treasure child. The third feature of the incident is that although we continued to be poisoned, crippled, and killed, in the tens of thousands, we never killed even a single person.

All three of these features are related to life. Cats died one after another. Birds died. People died. And yet though there might be times when we reduced our intake, we continued to eat the fish rumored to be the source of death. There were periods when we couldn't sell the fish we caught, but even these didn't last very long. You say it was because we didn't have anything else to eat, but that isn't the case. My family had rice paddies, fields, and woodlots. These generated food and cash, so we certainly could have survived without the fish. So why did we keep eating it? I believe that we fisherfolk were incapable of doubting any form of life, other than our fellow humans. We placed complete faith in life and received it with reverence and gratitude. We felt that Ebisu, the god of the sea, was sharing his bounty with us.

Beyond this, I must admit that I love fish. I feel that fish is unique among foods. Eating fish is part of my identity; I eat it with great happiness. My sisters say that just watching me eat makes them hungry. I even love the smell of fish; it is the smell of life.

Life being such a gift, death is a great moment. We treat it with as much ceremony as we do a birth. In the past, birth and death were central to our communal life. This reverence for life is the major reason that the victims of

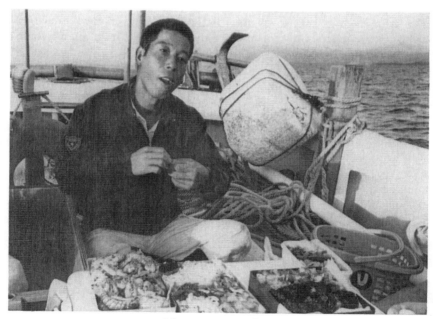

A feast on Masato's boat

Minamata disease did not kill anyone responsible for their condition. This doesn't mean we didn't hate Chisso. Who would not be angry if their children were crippled for life, their parents, brothers, and sisters killed? They killed thousands of us, but they suffered no casualties. To tell you the truth, I once thought of planting a bomb at Chisso. Now I'm glad I didn't disgrace our spiritual traditions in that way.

In our dialect we have a special expression, *nusari*. In the rest of Kumamoto Prefecture, they say *nosari*. *Nusari* means a gift, or a blessing. When we use this expression, we mean that destiny, everything that happens to us, is a gift. We must embrace it, whether good or bad. For example, when we have a good catch, we say, "We received a gift of many fish today." Or, let's say something bad happens. We might drop by the home of a friend or a village elder. They'll offer us some sake and let us talk it out. But in the end, their advice is always the same: "That, too, is *nusari*. You have to be patient." Or, "You have to embrace it." There is no room for argument. You accept what has happened, and you find that you are calm. You can return to your everyday life.

We have another expression, *gotagai*, which means "we're all in this together." This doesn't mean simply that we humans rely upon each other for our existence but that plants and animals are also partners in this life. *Gotagai* includes the sea, the mountains, everything. Human beings are part of the circle of *gotagai*; we owe our existence to the vast web of interrelationships that constitute life. Words like "settlement" and "compensation" are shallow terms, related only to human society. Of what meaning are these terms for the fish, the birds, the cats that were poisoned and killed by organic mercury? You can't compensate for their suffering and death with money. What about our rich intertidal and subtidal zones, our old-growth forests? How can you make up for their loss? You certainly cannot force them into a "settlement." I've been thinking about this for a long time.

The terms *nusari* and *gotagai* include reverence for, and a sense of humility toward, all life. We know that life is something larger than ourselves, a force before which we can only prostrate ourselves and pray. I think you can understand the three points I brought up earlier that characterize the Minamata incident: We continued to eat fish, we continued to have children, and we did not kill anyone. This philosophy of "life-ism" is all we need to stand up against the destructive aspects of modern civilization. There was no need to win a court battle. We had won before we began the proceedings.

Moyainaoshi, Moored Together Again

In the past we had no use for the word *shizen*, nature. It's only in the last twenty years or so that we've started to hear this word. Our lives were so immersed in nature there was no need to distinguish it. If people fell into a river or the sea, we would say that they had been sucked up by *garappa*, a water goblin. There are also many stories about people who have been tricked by foxes or *tanuki* (the raccoon dog, which resembles a badger). This is how our people described the powers of nature; on the one hand they warned us against its vagaries, and on the other they expressed feelings of closeness and affection.

There's a man in our village named Oshima, who loves to play *shogi* so much that a whole day will pass without his noticing. About thirty years ago, a turtle showed up at his house. Oshima offered him some sake and returned him to the ocean. The turtle continued to visit for the next three years, and during that time Oshima caught lots of fish. So even turtles understand the significance of returning a favor, his neighbors said. It's a famous story around these parts.

The tides differ according to the season. They change with a certain rhythm. When I'm in sync with that rhythm, I can read the sea, and the catch is good. But just let some other business call me away for three or four days, and I'm lost. It takes twice the time I was gone to regain my instincts. The rhythm of the tides is important not only for fishing but for all aspects of our lives. It is said that people are born at high tide and die at low tide. Women's bodily cycles are closely related to the tides and the moon. I remember my mother complaining that she much preferred the old lunar calendar. For a fisherwoman, it made much more sense than the solar calendar.

When I catch a lot of fish, I love the sea. But if I catch too many, I begin to get scared. To take fish is to take lives. If I take too many, I fear that I will pay with my own life. Other fishermen feel the same way. Night fishing is especially eerie. "Still alive!" I say thankfully when I awaken in the morning.

At least once a year there will be a boat with a large catch that doesn't return to port. My uneasiness is not mere superstition.

I suppose that these fears are designed to keep our greed in check. After all, we are dealing with living creatures. When we catch fish like *tai*, red snapper, that bring in a lot of money, we bleed the fish to keep them fresh. Each time I do this I feel apologetic toward the fish. I hear that many city people these days don't even know that fish have blood, but their blood is as red as ours.

When I'm fishing, the ocean is like a battleground. But there are also times when I am struck by its beauty. Sunset, sunrise, when the sea lies calm and still, or when the young leaves of spring suddenly burst open along the shore, I am so enchanted that I totally lose my sense of self. Men don't talk about such things, but I imagine other fishermen feel the same way.

Sadly, the ocean today is not the way I remember it. The water used to be so clear that you could spear sea cucumber thirty feet below the boat, but now you can't see down more than four or five feet. The biggest reason for this change is soil erosion. Ever since forests have been cleared for *mikan* orchards in the hills, topsoil has run down into the sea. Construction work, too, causes soil to run off. Places where the water was thirty feet deep when I was a child are now nearly filled in. One species of local coral is almost extinct.

Pesticides and chemical fertilizers have run into the sea as well. Seaweed that once grew in the tidal flats was poisoned. Its roots were destroyed, and the plants were buried in sand and mud. About twenty years ago people began fish farming, and high concentrations of waste spread through the water. It's hard to imagine that this area was once frequented by dolphins and whales.

When tourists come from the city they express their delight that such a beautiful coastal area remains in Japan, but they can't even imagine what this place used to be like. Our hills were covered with old-growth stands of pine, banyan, and laurel. Kelp beds called *moba*, which look like a meadow of seaweed stretching out to the sea, teemed with life. You would find the fry of horse mackerel and sea bream, as well as squid and shrimp. I remember the large crabs scuttling under our bare feet. When we put out our crab nets at high tide, we'd get so many that we could hardly pull them in. There were lots of other shellfish, too. It was mainly the women and children who went after the crabs and clams. Men would join in the hunt for octopus. Whether in the intertidal or in the deeper kelp forests, it was never hard to find something to eat. Now it all seems like a dream.

It was a bountiful sea. It was said that fish from the inland waters of the Shiranui Sea tasted much different from those caught in the outside waters.

People would say that once you had tasted *tachiuo*, a cutlass fish from the inland sea, you could never eat one from anywhere else. Not a trace of the old *moba* remain today. In their place, we have landfill and concrete. Needless to say, the catch has been reduced drastically. It's a tragedy. The magnitude of what we have traded for "progress" and "civilization" never ceases to astound me.

I remember quite vividly what the village and its people used to be like, and from the time of my nervous breakdown in 1985 that image has become increasingly important to me. The landscape speaks to me, working on my mind. This is the place where I was born and the place to which I will return. I'm not saying that I want to return to the way society was thirty or forty years ago. It had its good aspects, but it also had some very negative points, such as local conservatism. It would be a mistake to idealize the past. I would simply like to restore the deep wisdom at the root of our ancestors' daily lives and attempt to apply it to our current lifestyle. I am just the right age to bridge the old and the new.

In spite of waves of pollution and destruction, the Shiranui Sea and the mountains that rise up from its shores still embrace and nurture us. During

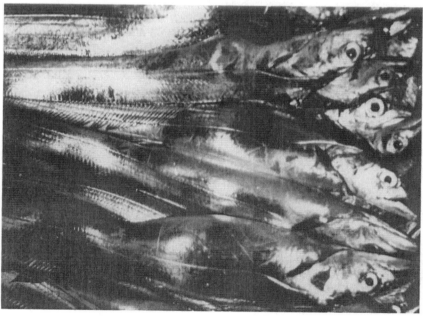

Masato's catch, tachiuo, a swordlike, scaleless silver fish
for which the Shiranui Sea is famous

my period of "madness" I realized that this is the world in which I must live. I have no need for the state. I have no need for a system that puts a price on human life and measures everything in financial terms. My life will be inseparable from the hills and sea. In this landscape it will be possible to communicate with the souls of those sacrificed by modern civilization. My native land still has the power to offer hints about how to live humanely.

In our village people kept busy year 'round. From winter to spring equinox we would collect seaweed, such as *wakame* and *hijiki*, and gather oysters. When the weather turned a bit warmer, it was time to hunt octopus. In the mountains we picked the fiddleheads of bracken, osmund, and silver-leaf ferns. We took only enough mountain greens for ourselves; we didn't sell them.

Spring was the season for sardine fry. During summer we'd catch the larger ones. After fall spawning we had another chance at the fry. Autumn nights were long. We spent every minute casting our nets and pulling them in. This was all done by hand, mind you. There were no motorized winches then, only pulleys.

Once they were back on shore, the crew would tell their neighbors to come get their shares of the catch. In the village there were households in which the father had died, leaving elderly parents, a wife, and children. We always made sure they had fish. Folks who commuted to work outside of the village and no longer fished came to get this special treat. Kids who helped out at the dock also received fish. We kept what we needed, but we gave away all the smaller fish. We all knew what our neighbors would be eating that night!

Of course, the sharing was never one-sided. Those who farmed would bring us sweet potatoes and vegetables. All of this sharing took place every day. It wasn't intended to be an equal exchange. If a household had nothing to give, no one considered it a problem. It was easy to give when the recipient was so grateful. Besides, we never thought of the fish as our own catch. It was a gift from Ebisu, the god of the sea.

It's not that we didn't have our quarrels. Everyone has his own likes and dislikes. By the next day, though, the argument would be forgotten. We all knew that we couldn't survive without cooperation. Intellectuals in the cities often refer to "autonomy" or "independence." If you used those words here in the village, people would laugh in your face. "What do you think you can do by yourself?" they would ask. They meant that we can't get by without depending on the sun and the moon and the help of our friends. Say someone wants to build a house. Villagers will go into the mountains, cut down the appropriate trees, and haul them to a sawmill. Once the logs have been cut into boards and pillars, friends will gather to haul them to the house site and begin building. People used to do everything themselves, from plastering walls to tiling roofs. But they couldn't have managed without a helping hand.

House building was a festive event. *Yoisho, yoisho,* people would chant, as they pulled on a rope to raise the ridgepole. Then someone would start to sing, and everyone would join in. Later, villagers would disguise themselves in costumes and dance through the streets. It was so much fun. There were always people who were good at singing and playing the *shamisen.* They took the lead. Our region is known for such improvised musical events, called *niwaka.*

The women were even wilder than the men. Often they would surprise the crowd with the erotic nature of their miming or dancing. Eroticism and drinking have always gone hand in hand. But while the men couldn't express themselves freely unless they drank, the women got drunk on the atmosphere itself. All the feelings they usually suppressed were now set free. It was an explosion of the soul, a form of release we all needed several times a year. Those wonderful singers, musicians, and dancers, so reserved in everyday life, now took center stage. Even the memories make me happy.

These must have been scenes typical of almost any village in the old days.

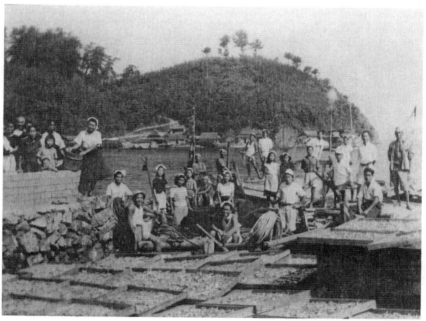

Members of a vibrant fishing community pose with their catch of sardines (Meshima, circa 1949).

Unfortunately, such festive occasions have almost disappeared today. It's been my dream to restore them, and so when our community hall was built, I suggested that we recreate such an event. At the ridgepole raising we asked the community chief to lead us in a song, and we asked the elementary school to help with the masquerade parade. I was hoping that if some of us took the lead in singing and dancing, others would join in, and to my delight the women were the first to step in the ring. Everyone looked for a chance to show off their talents. It was as if they had been waiting for this.

In the past, the year was marked by many ceremonies and rituals, such as weddings and funerals and boat launchings. I'm sure they contributed to the vibrant atmosphere of the village. People were bright-eyed and full of joyous laughter. Their smiles were different from the smiles you see today. Looking at the old photographs, you see that both men and women were healthy and happy. When I traveled to the Philippines and rediscovered those vibrant faces, I was filled with nostalgia.

In our village you would never let a visitor go without offering him or her a meal. "Let's chat," was the common invitation. If you hadn't seen someone in a while, you would be especially insistent that the person stay to have a drink and eat with you. If it was a guest from outside the village, we would prepare many different dishes in advance and go out of our way to make sure he or she had a good time. This kind of hospitality hasn't been forgotten today, and I feel proud of it.

In the past we had neither television nor highways. We didn't get much news overland. But we were far from being a closed and isolated community. All the coastal villages were connected by the same inland sea.

In the old days we never locked anything. Our door didn't have a key. The shouts of couples fighting carried to the next house, and everyone knew what was going on with their neighbors. Men didn't dominate their households. Women were just as aggressive, hurling pots and pans and whatever they could get their hands on. No one interfered. We had a saying, "When the sun sets, the southerly wind calms, and couples stop fighting." So, despite these little spats, the community remained united. I see it as a "spiritual community." But gradually a materialistic society began to erode this spiritualism and transform the village.

The school system played a major role in destroying the traditional ways of the community. Adults didn't anticipate this. To many parents, school was just a playground for their kids. We used to skip classes and go up into the mountains. We did this so often that the teacher finally visited our families. I remember my mother scolding me when I came home. "Playing hooky again! Don't you know you make your teachers worry!" Evidently the teachers were worried about their position, not about us. And my mother was worried about them. No one in the village took this type of education seriously. Parents thought that as long as their children didn't inconvenience others, it didn't matter how they decided to live. No one ever told me to study. Can you imagine that happening today?

In the past, our community had two faces: one looking outward and one looking inward. The villagers' attitude toward education is one example. They would say one thing to the teachers and hold a different view at home. Their attitude toward Buddhist temples is similar. Most villagers identify with the Nishi-Honganji sect of Buddhism. But they are indifferent to this religion except during funerals. To them, it is "funeral Buddhism." The priests, for their part, wouldn't think of lending a hand to help a sick parishioner. Their indifference persisted through forty years of Minamata disease. The villagers were not disturbed. They continued to support the temples but did not place their trust in established religion. We might compare the situation to schoolchildren listening politely to a boring lecture. Beyond the pale of Buddhism were local gods like Ebisu and the gods of the hills. These were the gods important to the villagers' daily lives. And at the foundation of all the villagers did was the human soul.

Perhaps the community began to decline when its two faces became

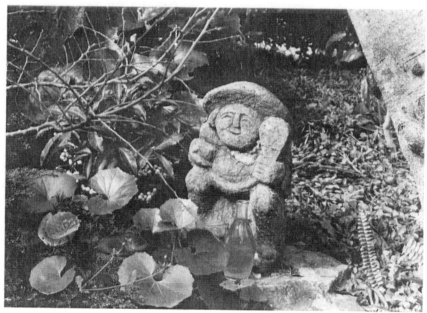

*A small stone image of the god of the rice paddies, in Masato's garden.
Before the image are offerings of beer and sake.*

blurred. In other words, villagers lost their ability to distinguish between the outside and the inside. Together with the influx of goods and information from outside, something of the village left. As we lost our culture, we believed that we were becoming "cultured."

Even so, I can still detect some of the community spirit. For example, a few years ago an NHK film crew came to the village. When they were done, we held a barbecue for them at the community hall. Villagers gathered to drink with them. All of a sudden I noticed that the entire NHK crew had left while we were all still in our seats, drinking. Apparently they had gotten drunk and retreated to their van. I got really mad. We had thrown a party in their honor, and they left without even thanking us. The villagers tried to calm me. They assured me that they were not offended, that they really didn't care. It was then that I saw the community still existed; here were my neighbors, telling me that they understood. Those NHK people were from outside, they seemed to be saying. They didn't share our customs and feelings, so it would be best to let them go their own way. In this instance I found that the communal tradition of maintaining two faces was still alive.

For young people who have no experience of communal life, it's hard to find the road home. But I want to let them know that there is a place to which they may return. It's true that even a village community is a kind of system. But the "spiritual community" of which I speak lacks the size and complexity of national society. Rather, it exists close at hand in our daily lives. It is a cyclical system, based on nothing more complex than catching fish and eating it.

The spiritual community is like an old-fashioned country stew, in which each person has a different face, physique, character, and age. Some would be disabled. But regardless of their characteristics, all would have valuable roles to play. No one would be dispensable. In such a society there would be no discrimination. To acknowledge each other's differences is to acknowledge our essential equality.

We have an expression, *moyai*, which I hold close to my heart. You folks from the city probably aren't familiar with this term, so let me explain. It comes from the verb *moyau*, which means "to tie two boats together," or "to moor a boat to a piling." For instance, when we fished for sardines, two boats of the same size would drag a net between them. This was called a *moyai* net, and the boats were called *moyai* boats. If a storm should blow up while we were fishing, we would tie our boat together with another and head for port. This, too, is called *moyau*. The other boat didn't necessarily belong to an acquaintance. It might be a boat from Amakusa, for example. As we headed for port we would talk about our fishing villages, how the fish were running, and so on. This gave fishermen a valuable opportunity to exchange news and information. Even in fair weather, three or four boats might tie up together to discuss the tides, talk about where the fish were, and make sure we weren't encroaching on someone else's fishing spot.

Moyai began as a fishing term, but it has been applied to other aspects of our daily lives. For example, someone might say, "I'm going to the temple today, so why don't we *moyau,* go together?" It implies that a small group of people will go somewhere and also return together. Villagers enjoy going places together.

Today, *moyai* holds a special significance for me. Over the past forty years modern technology has seeped into our region, and we have embraced it with open arms. In my own life I have experienced extreme highs and lows. But now that I am on my feet again, I want to return to the place I belong. Of course, the journey home requires a lot of courage. To go alone would be too lonely. So, what if I were to call out, "*Moyoute kaeroo!*" "Let us moor together again. Let us return together."

Minamata is a paradoxical place. On the one hand, it's a place where life was destroyed, year after year. Everyone knows this. But there are few who see the other side of the picture. Minamata is also a place where life per-

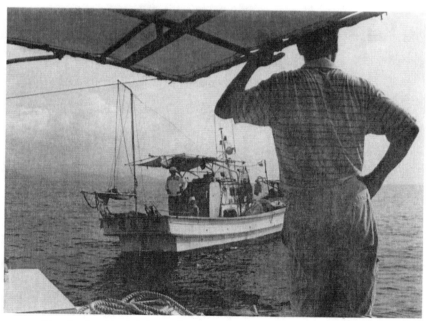

Moyai—drawing their boats close together, Masato and another fisherman share news on the fishing grounds.

sisted, year after year. Much of our natural world survived. Because it is a place that endured so much suffering, it is also a place where people have earnestly explored the meaning of life. When I was young I didn't understand Ishimure Michiko's expression, "*kugai jodo,* paradise in the sea of sorrow." But as I grow older, I've come to understand what she means. This bitter sea, our human lives, or the sea of sorrow, our inland sea, may also be seen as a paradise where life endures and is celebrated.

We tend to interpret life through dualistic thinking. Some people say, "An evil spirit descended on Minamata." But in what sense do they use these words, "evil spirit"? Are we contrasting evil and injustice with good and justice? Someone asked me recently, "What is the origin of the tragedy that befell Minamata?" At a loss for an answer, I said, "The back of the Buddha." But, as I think about it, it's true. Good and evil are two expressions of the same thing. It is true that an evil force descended on our birthplace, the Shiranui Sea. But this can also be a place where gods descend. We must make it so.

When I embarked on a new life in 1985, I gave myself a new name, Kaizan Kochidomari. *Kaizan* means "mountains and sea," while *Kochidomari* means "eastern anchorage." This is the name of my hamlet. My name reflects my

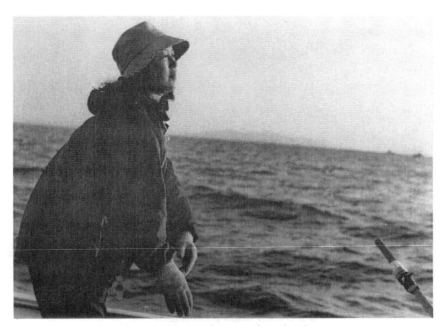

Masato's wife, Sawako, at work on their boat

natural and social surroundings. This is where I was born, and here I will die. The name of my study, this little outbuilding where I've been telling you my life story, is "Yuuan," "a hut where the soul drifts freely." The scroll hanging on the wall behind me commemorates the launching ceremony for my wooden boat, *Tokoyo*, "The Eternal World." The calligraphy over the entrance is something I wrote a few years ago on New Year's Day:

> Embraced by the mountains and sea
> Ego dissolves; self and landscape are one.

I have already selected the Buddhist name by which I will be known after I die. It is Yuuantei Ooutsuke, "The great fool of the house of 'Yuuan.'" I have even prepared a will. Although most people in Japan today are cremated, I have requested that my family bury me in the ground. Place three stones over me to mark the spot, I wrote, and at the funeral please have a wild party and enjoy yourselves.

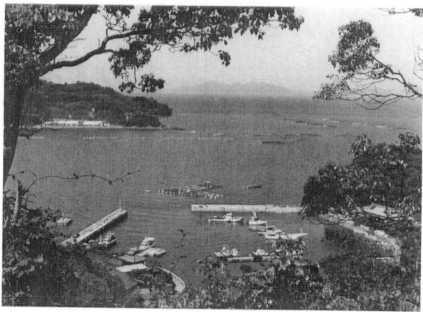

A view from the hill overlooking Masato's house (bottom left) and the hamlet of Kochidomari

Epilogue

Oiwa Keibo

The most appropriate word for the unusual nature of my encounter with Ogata Masato is *en*, a word of special significance for him. *En* refers to a mysterious power, or karmic force, that connects two people or establishes a relationship between a person and certain phenomena or events. It was the people from a Buraku community in Fukuoka Prefecture who introduced Masato to me. The Buraku people, or Burakumin, still carry the stigma of the outcaste status held by their ancestors.

It was April 30, 1994. My Burakumin friends drove me from Fukuoka to Minamata, a little fishing village in Kumamoto Prefecture. It was a beautiful spring day, and the ocean was calm and flat like a mirror. The scent of *mikan* blossoms filled the air. By this time, the name "Minamata" was known all over the world. However, it wasn't through the Minamata issue that I had come to meet Masato. Rather, it was through Masato that I gained an intimate view of the world of the Minamata incident.

Earlier that March, I had visited F-*san*'s family at their home in Chikushino City, Fukuoka. F-*san*, a leader of the Burakumin community, is a municipal welfare officer. He has long sought to bridge his Buraku community with the communities in Minamata, to create mutual support networks, and to collaborate in the search for alternative lifestyles. F-*san* met Masato when Masato was leading the Minamata struggle, and they became close friends.

When I expressed my desire to visit Masato, F-*san* immediately offered to accompany me. He believes that Ogata's message reaches far beyond the limits of Minamata and that Buraku people in particular, as an oppressed minority, have much to learn from his personal struggle. "Golden Week," a week incorporating several national holidays, had just begun on April 29. This day also marks the late Showa emperor's birthday, now ironically called Green

177

Day. F's children had the day off from school, so the whole family packed up in a van with me and drove from Fukuoka to Minamata. On the way, the family told me how much they enjoyed their visits to the Minamata region. Before they met Masato, they had had a bleak image of Minamata; they associated it with tragedy and suffering. But the Minamata they found was a warm and lively community, extending from wooded hills to the shimmering sea.

As we approached Masato's village, Meshima, I noticed how the mountains and hills suddenly dive into the ocean, leaving almost no flat land for farming. F-san's family told me that this is typical landscape for the area, which partly explains the heavy reliance on fishing and the unstable nature of the local economy.

"When Minamata folk say they eat fish, they mean something quite different than we would," F-san said. "For us, eating fish refers to eating a piece of fish as part of a meal. We might eat fish a few times a week. For them, it is almost the whole meal, every day. It's their staple diet." I could understand from F-san's explanation how susceptible these fisherfolk would be to mercury poisoning.

Masato greeted us in front of his home. A few steps from his house, across a narrow street, is a concrete breakwater. Masato, a handsome, weathered, slender man, wore the traditional blue working clothes of a monk. He seemed to emanate strength, yet when he broke into a huge friendly smile I saw his other side.

He invited us to a small one-room study and guesthouse that he had named "Yuuan," "a hut where the soul drifts freely." Here our discussion continued for the next four hours over tea, beer, and Masato's beloved local liquor, *shochu*. It was a place to which I would return again and again in the years to come, to sit for days conversing with him. Masato's words had unusual conviction and power. Even when he referred to his period of "insanity," he was articulate and logical. He said there had been many times when he was tempted to take his life, as if amazed, even now, that he had come through.

"In the time of my father and grandfather, people's words were full of spirit. At community gatherings, Father and Grandfather didn't even have to speak. Their presence was so strong and eloquent that a single word sparked like lightning and resounded like thunder." Then he added, "But look around now. Television vomits empty words and hollow noise." When Masato spoke about his forefathers, who today rest just over the top of the hill looking down on his house, his words bore the dignified air of myth. "Now, I understand that my grandparents were *dojin*, a bunch of aborigines, people belonging to a place. Then, one day, the System, capitalism and modernization, came upon them."

Our first conversation drew to a close as F's children, tired of playing with crabs along the shore, waited close by, anxious to leave. But as we stood out by a rocky incline, saying farewell, Masato talked a bit more. The sun was comfortably warm. Looking down on the waterline, Masato pointed out that high tide would bring the water right up to where we now stood. He added, "When the ocean was calm, I felt so many times like stepping out onto the water and walking along the path of the moonlight. I felt so sure that I could make it to the end." As we bid farewell, I knew that I would be coming back. His story began taking shape in my mind, a story that deserved to be told.

When I first apologized for my ignorance about the Minamata incident, he said without changing his expression, "Factual knowledge isn't important to me anyway." But later, when I started interviewing him for the book, I immediately found myself surrounded by facts. I often wondered if I was the right person to write this book, but the joy of being with Masato always overshadowed my worries. Interviewing him was always exciting and dynamic, with each of us asking questions, discussing, and arguing. He seemed as curious about me as I was about him. For hours at a time we sat in "Yuuan" on the wood floor, facing each other across the *irori*, a fire pit. In summer a refreshing ocean breeze blew across the deck and through the open window where we sat. In winter, the stars sparkled. Sometimes a powderlike snow covered the garden. I would lean over the glowing coals to keep warm as hot steam shot out of the black iron kettle beside me.

Masato's wife, Sawako, served one dish after another. One spring afternoon the menu included slices of raw wild-caught *tai*, red snapper; *nimono*, stewed fish and vegetables, fish head included; *fuka*, boiled shark meat with a vinegar and miso sauce; *ika*, raw squid; *namako*, sea cucumber with vinegar; deep-fried *hamo*, sea eel, and fish cakes. I was always impressed with Masato's appetite, but my own appetite at his house was also incredible. My favorite dish was fresh *tachiuo*, a long swordlike, scaleless, silver fish, a specialty of the region. Fresh *aji*, horse mackerel, and squid had an amazing sweetness I had never tasted in the city. This variety of fresh fish, everyday fare to the local resident, was a real treat for a city person.

Masato is a "good drinker" of *shochu*, in the tradition of his father and grandfather. Our long discussions were interrupted only when one or both of us would go outside to stand by the water's edge and relieve ourselves. Masato once told me that one of the main problems he encounters when visiting the city is that he cannot urinate outside. "Peeing in a toilet is just not the same," he said.

Masato and Sawako have taken me fishing with them many times. Here,

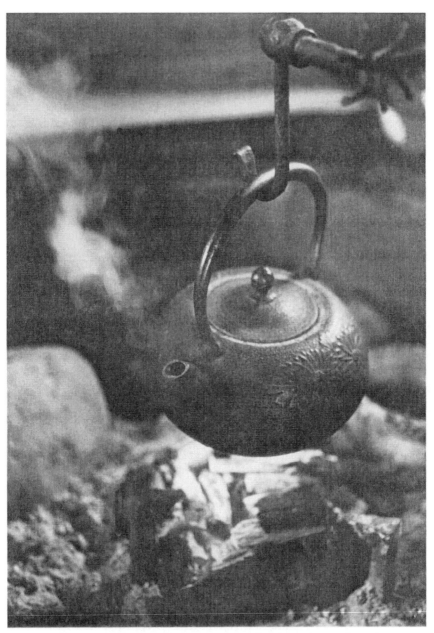

Inside "Yuuan" an iron kettle steams over burning charcoal on a winter day.

in the calm waters of the Shiranui Sea, it is still common to see a small boat with a couple working side by side. Masato jokingly says, "Couples here fight a lot, but they know how to make up quickly so that the next day's work is not missed." For *tachiuo* fishing we would leave the house a few hours before sunset. First, Masato would determine where to set the nets. After the place was found, Sawako would begin dropping the weighted nets with rhythmic precision. With a triangular hood covering her face, she picked up the weighted ends, throwing them one by one into the water as Masato steered. Finally the long net was set at the bottom of the sea, and we opened our picnic dinner on the boat, watching the slow descent of the sun. By the time they started pulling in the nets, it was dark, and small squid gathered around the boat, attracted by the light.

On some of my trips Masato and I would go to Minamata City and walk around the reclaimed land of Minamata Bay. Walking in a forest overlooking the reclaimed land, we discovered a grove of old banyan trees with roots wrapped about huge boulders. We knew instantly that this was an ancient place of worship. On our next visit, we were drawn to the forest by singing voices and festive sounds. There we encountered a group of fifty or sixty people, mostly elderly, sitting on the ground partying. It was a festival in honor

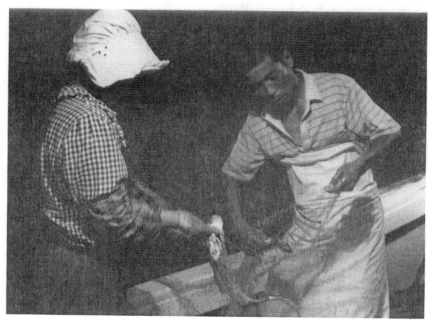

Masato and Sawako fish on a summer night.

of a god represented by a small stone statue. It was a mountain god, they explained, who had been washed downstream by the river and ended up at the shore. Each time it washed down, local residents would return the god to its place in the hills, but eventually it would find its way back to shore. Finally it was decided that the god must belong by the ocean. Now it sits on a small hill on the edge of the banyan grove, looking down over Minamata Bay and nearby Koiji Island.

On another occasion we strolled along the edge of the reclaimed land, stopping to admire each of the little statues carved by Masato and his friends. They all look toward the island and into the ocean beyond. On yet another visit we walked over the hill down to the neighboring hamlet of Kyodomari, where many of Masato's relatives live. There we visited his nephew Tatsuzumi, who was born with Minamata disease. I watched Masato and Tatsuzumi play *shogi*, Japanese chess. Tatsuzumi, with his one arm permanently curled close to his body, would lean far over the chessboard as if talking to the pieces as he moved them. After beating Masato, he challenged me to a round. I beat him. That's how we became friends. Not many words were exchanged during this visit, but Masato and I were very happy walking back. I remember most clearly his peaceful and relaxed laughter while visiting with Tatsuzumi.

Masato's words were new and refreshing. There was a strange and almost mysterious clarity to his ideas that I have rarely experienced. I have wondered where this clarity comes from. Two responses from overseas to Masato's story might provide hints.

When I visited Masato for the first time, I was in the midst of researching a book I was writing with David Suzuki, a renowned Canadian biologist, broadcaster, and environmental activist. The book was eventually published as *The Japan We Never Knew* (in the United States, *The Other Japan*), and it dealt with Japan's peace, environmental, and minority issues. David couldn't find time to visit Masato with me, so I sent my notes to him after my visit. His response was immediate and enthusiastic. First, David responded to Masato's critical ideas on "compensation," referring to his own experience with the Japanese–Canadian redress movement. From the 1970s in the United States, and from the 1980s in Canada, the redress movement had called for a government apology for the forced relocation and incarceration of Japanese and of Americans and Canadians of Japanese ancestry during World War II. Initiated by the *sansei*, or third-generation Japanese, the movement pointed out how this "internment" had violated human and constitutional rights and had been based on racial discrimination. The official excuse of "military necessity" for this incarceration clearly masked its racist origin.

In 1988, the governments of both countries signed a settlement that apologized to the survivors and provided monetary compensation to underscore the sincerity of the apology. David had lent his influence to the movement, declaring that this settlement would provide a precedent for other movements to address past wrongs. David declined to accept the settlement money, but he felt it offered a model for Indians seeking justice in North America.

In 1988 I was living in Canada and participating in the redress movement. I witnessed the way in which monetary compensation caused deep divisions among citizens of Japanese descent. David shares Masato's view that "when you receive money, something important is lost forever." Masato's efforts to recover his sense of self—his identity as a human being and not just as a victim and a patient—struck a chord with David. Moreover, David, one of the leading figures in the world environmental movement, appreciated Masato's view that what is lost forever in exchange for money is "ourselves as a part of nature." In scientific and technological civilization, Mother Earth has been relegated to a "resource," and everything on it has been given a price tag. Like Masato, David believes that this is the wellspring of the worldwide environmental crisis.

In November 1995, I helped organize a conference in Vancouver called the Canada–Japan Minority Forum. At this conference, I had the opportunity to speak about Masato and the Minamata incident. The strongest reaction to my talk came from indigenous (Native Canadian) members of the audience. One of them was Loretta Todd, a Cree filmmaker and conference panelist. She told me of her interest in making a film about Masato, and later she wrote a proposal for this project. From her experience with reservation life, it must have been easy to understand Masato's concepts of spiritual incarceration as a result of the settlement process. Just as Native North Americans have been alienated from nature and their cultural traditions, left jobless, and forced to become dependent on the state welfare system, the community of Minamata has been distorted through the settlement process. The social problems on reservations—including poverty, alcoholism, domestic violence, crime, and high suicide rates—add to the frustration of Native people. Often government-sponsored assistance programs have ended up discouraging self-governance and reinforcing a system of economic and political dependency. Both groups have asked for compensation but ended up more dependent than when they started.

But, as Loretta depicts in her films, there are new movements toward true self-government, even in the midst of social crisis. In many places throughout North America, Native people are seriously discussing the necessity to break the circle of dependency. In her proposal for the film on Masato, Loretta wanted to put the Minamata situation in this context. "The crisis of society is also a crisis of self. Let us return to where we belong," said Masato. Needless to say, Masato's refrain, "We are all Native people who cannot be separated from the ocean, mountains, rivers, grass, and trees," is as familiar to indigenous people as a mother's lullaby.

Masato loves to play with words. At the end of a lecture delivered in Tokyo, he said, "I believe that I will return to Tokyo to meet you again. It would be auspicious if you were to give me, not *shien*, but *goen*." In this context, *shien* means support, and *goen* refers to a karmic force that brings people together. His reference to *shien* resonated with the audience, who were mostly Minamata-movement activists and had grown used to hearing about "supporters" and "victims." Instead, Masato was calling for a more creative and spiritual relationship among the people of Minamata, and between them and outsiders offering support. *Goen* also means "five yen," and *shien* is "four yen," implying the greater value of *goen*. In fact, this is part of a rhyme Masato made up in which five yen becomes four yen, which becomes three yen, and on down the line as the moral value is degraded. In this short pun the complex thoughts of someone whose personal history is entangled with the history of the Minamata incident are revealed and summarized.

On another occasion, talking about his plan to place stone images on the reclaimed land in Minamata Bay, Masato told me, "My original idea was to place uncarved stones there. Why stones? I want to express my intention and will." In Japanese, both the word for "stone" and the word for "intention, will" are pronounced *ishi*. He continued, "Also, I had been thinking of the fact that Tanaka Shozo, who sided with the peasants in the Ashio copper-mine pollution incident, had with him only a little bag with tissue and a few stones when he died." Tanaka Shozo (1841–1913), the leading figure in Japan's first great environmental struggle, is one of Masato's heroes.

Looking back to his past, Masato realized that his leaving home at a young age constituted a spiritual departure, analogous to becoming a monk. The *kanji*, or Chinese characters, for "leaving home," when reversed, read "spiritual departure." During his period of "madness" Masato's mind was bombarded with puns, allowing him to look at reality from many different perspectives. Conversely, his current use of word play is a way of practicing and reviewing this period of "madness." I do not claim to understand his "madness"; I can only imagine what it was like. When I do so, I like to compare it to a vision quest in the Native American tradition. In a vision quest a young person on the verge of becoming a mature member of society would go into the wilderness for days without eating, and would endure a series of ordeals. Finally, overcome with hunger and fatigue, the youth would experience a vision, which would direct the person's adult life. It is tempting to look at Masato as a shaman who has appeared on the margin of contemporary Japanese life. His story reminds me of the latent possibilities of an area that has been sealed off by modern intellect, labeled "madness," ignored as delusional, and despised as an artifact of the "primitive mind."

The world is interconnected. But this connection doesn't simply refer to physical connections. What has been revealed to Masato, and what he has been trying to share with us, is the interconnectedness of meanings. Ours is not just the physical world, it is the world of meaning and spirit. As a contemporary shaman, Masato is warning us of our total separation from the meaningful world. But he also points to a solution. It is a return to a spiritual world on Earth, in which everyone and everything has a place. It is a world in which life is respected, worshipped, and celebrated.

Index

activism on Minamata disease: early, 8–9; goals of, 12; and objectification, 150; Ogata and, 77, 79–86, 81f, 86f. *See also* Minamata movement
Akazaki Satoru, 105
Amakusa Islands, 23f, 25
amanatsu, 33
ami, 33
amphetamines, 67–68
ancestors. *See* deceased; spirits
apology for Minamata disease, 12
Ariake Sea mercury poisoning incident, 10
Ashikita Mountains, 109
ashinaka sandals, 114
Association of Original Vow, 122

bearing witness, 104, 107, 109–16
boat launching ceremony, 17–21, 105
boat spirit, 37
bora, 33
Boy's Day, 71, 115
Buddha, 154
Buddha statues, 121–24, 124f, 129, 130f, 136, 182
Buddhism, attitudes toward, 171
Buraku people (Burakumin), 84, 125n3, 177–78

cadmium poisoning, 10
Canada: industrial pollution incidents in, 4f, 13–14, 80; traditional peoples in, 182–84
carp streamers, 71f, 115
cats, and Minamata disease, 1, 5, 131f
certification process for Minamata disease, 9, 143–44, 147
chemical fertilizers, 166
children: and Minamata disease, 54–55; and sit-in at Chisso, 113–14
Chisso Corporation, 1–3, 16n43, 46f, 110f–111f, 116; and compensation payments, 144–45; employment by, 12; Ogata family and, 115–16; Ogata Masato and, 101, 104, 109–16, 112f; pollution by, 2–3, 6, 11; protests of, 69, 74, 75f, 109–16, 112f; response to investigation, 789; rioting at, 46–47; working conditions in, 3
Citizens' Council for Minamata Disease Countermeasures, 8–9
civilization, Ogata on, 13, 122, 138, 164, 167
class: and fishing, 34; Ogata on, 153
closure, 11, 146–48, 154–55; resistance to, 118, 122, 156
Colligan-Taylor, Karen, 1–16
communism, 57
compassion, 12
compensation, 144–45; effects of, 153–54; meaning of, 153; and Minamata move-

ment, 145; Ogata on, 148, 150; Oiwa on, 183
concentration camps, 130–31
Concert for Ten Thousand People, 117–19
connection: activism and, 150; with life, 164; Ogata and, 99–100; Oiwa on, 177, 185; with Tatsutzumi, 161
contentment, 91–92
cooperation, 168–69
crew of *utasebune*, 137–41
cutlass, 26, 167, 167f, 179

death, Ogata on, 44, 163–64, 175
deceased: ceremony for, at Minamata Tokyo Exposition, 140–41; communication with, 129; connections with, 100; and transmission of souls, 156
demon fire festival, 51–52
Detsuki, 5
Devil's Island, 100
dolphins, 31
drinking, 31, 38, 169, 178–79
dualism, 174

East Germany, 133
Ebisu-*san*, 35–37, 36f, 163, 168
economy, 10
education. *See* school
Eleventh Day Festival, 37
employees of Chisso: and sit-in, 111, 114–15; working conditions of, 3
en, 177
Environment Agency, 10, 80
environmentalism: European conference on, 132–34; Japan and, 10–11; in Minamata, 12; Ogata on, 13; politics and, 84; traditions and, 37
Environmental Protection Agency (US), 16n43
Eternal World, Ishimure on, 18
Europe, Ogata in, 130–34
evil, Ogata on, 174
Ezuno family, 7–8

factual knowledge, Ogata on, 179
farming, 33, 54, 168

festivals, 169–70, 172
Final Settlement (Compromise Settlement, *Wakai Kyotei*), 11, 135–36, 146–48; Kawamoto and, 152–53
fishing (industry): balance in, 165–66; compensation payments for, 3, 7; and cycles, 172; farmers and, 33, 54; F-*san* on, 178; Minamata disease panic and, 73–74; Ogata and, 73–74, 102; status of, 88; techniques in, 26; traditions of, 33–38
fixed-shore-net fishing, 26
foods, traditional, 168
forests, 34, 166
forgiveness, Ogata on, 155
Fruit Growers Association of Minamata Patient Families, 88
F-*san*, 177–78
funerals, 44–45
future, Ogata on, 156–57

gago, 43
gangsters, 63–65, 67, 70, 82
Germany, 130–34
Gibbs, Lois Marie, 16n46
gizzard shad, 33
go-between, 87
god of rice paddies, 171f
gods: of mountain, 181–82; of rice paddies, 171f. *See also* spirits
goen, 184
gotogai, 164
government. *See* Japanese government; local government
Grassy Narrows, Ontario, Canada, 4f
green tourism, 12

halfbeak, 33
Hannaga Kazumitsu, 7–8
Harada Masuzumi, 6
hard work, 31–32, 65, 89–90
harmonious development, 133
Higa Yasuo, 122
Hirohito, emperor of Japan, 3
Hiroshima, 138
Hitomi (niece), 58–60

Holocaust, 130–32
hongan, 121–22
Hongan no Kai, 122
hosho. See compensation
Hosokawa Hajime, 5–7, 9
Hosokawa Morihiro, 117, 119
house-building, 168–69
human nature: activism and, 150; versus blame, 146; Ogata on, 138
Hyakken Harbor, 6

Ikawa, teacher, 53
Ikenoshiri, 127f
industrialization: increase in, 10; Ogata on, 122
industrial pollution, 10, 13–14, 75; in Canada, 4f, 13–14, 80; Chisso and, 2–3, 6, 11; in Europe, 133; left-wing politics and, 84
intuition, 34–35
irori, 179, 180f
Ishimure Michiko, 7–8, 10, 19f, 17–21, 174; meaning of name, 97
Itai itai disease, 10

Japanese government: and Chisso payments, 9–10; and clean-up, 11; and compensation, 11–12, 145, 153; dealing with past, 129–30; economic policy of, 2, 11–12; and environmentalism, 132–34; and Final Settlement, 146–47; protests of, 80–81, 81f, 86f; and reclaimed land, 121; response to Minamata disease, 86, 143–50; and responsibility, 146
jimotogaku, 12

Kagoshima, 84
Kaizan Kochidomari, 174–75. *See also* Ogata Masato
Kanemi Corporation, 84, 125n2
Kawamoto Teruo, 4f, 4–5, 81f; background of, 85; in Canada, 80; death of, 151–52; and Final Settlement, 152–53; meaning of name, 97; and Minamata movement,

10, 152–53; Ogata and, 85, 93, 95–96, 151–52
kelp beds, 166
ken-ri, 119
kibyo, 5
Kina Shokichi, 122–23
kioku, 1–2
kiroku, 1–2
Kobayashi, 139
kogai gannen, 10
Koiji Island, 123, 123f
koinobori, 71f, 115
konoshiro, 33
Kosaki Tatsuzumi, 8, 20–21, 58, 160f, 160–61, 182
kugai jodo, 174
Kumamoto City, 62–65, 67–70
Kumamoto Prefecture, 144
Kumamoto University, 68; Hospital, 40; School of Medicine, 6
Kyodomari, 162f, 182

laborers, 2–3. *See also* employees of Chisso
left-wing politics, and industrial pollution, 84
Liberal Democratic Party, 57
life: connection with, 164; Ogata on, 159–64, 168–69; Oiwa on, 185
litigation process, 9
local government: Kawamoto and, 152; Ogata and, 80, 103–4; protests of, 117–19
loneliness: Kawamoto and, 151–52; Ogata and, 96–97, 113
Love Canal, 16n46

madness: character for, 102; Ogata and, 95–102, 184–85; Tatsutzumi and, 161
Maruzen Sekiyu Corporation, 3
matsu, 161
mejiro, 51
mercury, 1, 3, 6, 8, 11, 133
Meshima, 25, 74
Minamata area: changes in, 12; map, x; Ogata on, 173–74; population of, 3–4, 12

Minamata disease, 1; congenital, 7, 159–61; continuing effects of, 122, 133–34; court decisions on, 75, 86; first appearance of, 5–6; investigation of, 6–7; reactions to, 5–6, 21n1, 54–55, 58–59; responsibility for, 12, 143–50; third outbreak of, 73–74, 125n1

Minamata Disease Certification Applicant's Council, 10, 75; Ogata and, 79–80, 85–86

Minamata disease patients: attitudes of, 59–60; and Final Settlement, 147–48, 150; message to, 111–12; and *nobotoke*, 121–22; number of, 4; Ogata Fukumatsu, 39–41; Ogata Masato, 55, 88; support for, 83

Minamata Fishermen's Association, 74

Minamata movement, 79, 83–84, 88, 150, 154–55; banner of, 83*f*; factions in, 9, 57–58; goals of, 144–45; Kawamoto and, 152–53; Ogata and, 87, 91–93, 155, 162–63

Minamata Municipal Hospital, 44

Minamata Tokyo Exposition, 136, 138, 140–41

Miyako Islands, 122–23

moba, 166

mochi, 51

modernization, Ogata on, 138, 153

money: and Minamata movement, 145; Ogata on, 43–47, 88, 97, 99–100, 119, 148, 153–54; versus responsibility, 154; Suzuki on, 183

moyai, 172–73, 173*f*

moyainaoshi, 165–75

mullet, 26

Nagasaki, 84, 138

nakodo, 87

namasu, 37

Native Canadians, 183–84

nature, Ogata on, 135, 165

neko-no-haka, 131*f*

New Tokyo International Airport, 84

New Year's Day, 33, 37

Nichigetsu-maru, 136–41, 139*f*

Niigata mercury poisoning incident, 8

Nippon Chisso Hiryo (Japan Nitrogen Fertilizer), 2

niwaka, 169

nobotoke, 121–24, 124*f*, 129, 130*f*, 136, 182

Noguchi Shitagau, 2

nusari, 164

Obon festival, 33, 37

ocean, 121, 166–67

octanol, 3

octopus, 33

Ogata family, 21, 25–27, 45*f*, 49–52; and activism, 79, 87; and compensation payments, 148; and education, 53; and father's illness, 40; grave of, 50*f*; and lawsuit, 57–58; and Masato's return, 73; oldest brother in, 61; oldest sister in, 61; and Tatsutzumi, 161; and *Tokoyo*, 105; uncle in, 87

Ogata Fukumatsu (father), 6, 8, 29–32, 30*f*, 92, 111; and family, 25, 49; funeral of, 44–45, 45*f*; grave of, 50*f*; intuition of, 34–35; and Minamata disease, 39–41, 44–45; and soul transmission, 156

Ogata Mamiko, 116

Ogata Masato, 45*f*, 107*f*, 181*f*; and application for certification, 79, 96, 103, 155–56; arrests of, 81–82; background of, 1, 25; children of, 91, 97, 115–16; and compensation payments, 148, 150; and father's death, 40–41, 44–45, 49; getting lost, 43–44; health of, 55, 88, 115, 135–36; Ishimure and, 17–21; jobs of, 64–65, 67–70, 88–90; leaving home, 61–65, 67–70; leaving movement, 91–93; marriage of, 87–90; meaning of name, 97; nervous breakdown, 95–102, 184–85; Oiwa on, 177–85; philosophy of, 156, 159–75; in protests, 81*f*, 86*f*, 117–19; questioning by, 91–93, 98; return home, 73–77; sit-in at Chisso, 109–16, 112*f*; and testing, 40–41, 99; voyage to Tokyo, 136–41; walk to reclaimed land, 134–35

Ogata (mother), 25–27, 45*f*; background of, 33–34; and family, 49; and father's illness, 41; and movement, 91–92, 103; Ogata and, 43–44, 54; philosophy of, 159, 161–62

Ogata Sawako (wife), 87, 91, 157*f*, 174*f*, 179–81, 181*f*; and breakdown, 97, 101; and Chisso Corporation, 115–16; and compensation payments, 148; and protest, 117–19; and *Tokoyo*, 107–8; and withdrawal of application, 103

Oita, 84

Oiwa Keibo, 177–85

Oki, 25–27

Okinawa, 122–23

opossum shrimp, 33

Oshima, 165

pachinko, 67

Pacific Ocean, sailing in, 140

past, connections with, 100

PCBs, 84, 125n2

pesticides, 166

Philippines, 10, 170

plastic, boats, 17–18, 104

Poland, 130–34

police, Ogata and, 43–44, 69, 81–82, 112–13

politics: and environmental movements, 84; Kawamoto and, 93; Ogata and, 57, 67–69, 77

pollution. *See* industrial pollution

polychlorinated biphenyls (PCBs), 84, 125n2

polyvinyl chloride (PVC), 3

progress, Ogata on, 138, 167

purse seining, 26

PVC, 3

Ramon Magsaysay Prize, 10

reclaimed land, 12, 124, 132*f*, 135*f*, 181–82, 184; government concert on, 117–19; in Nagasaki, 84; Ogata on, 119, 121–24; in Tokyo, 141; walk to, 134–35

reconciliation centers, 12

red snapper, 26, 74, 166

religion: and fishing, 35–37; villagers and, 171, 171*f*. *See also* gods; spirits

resistance: to civilization, 164; to closure, 118, 122, 156; by villagers, 171–72

responsibility: Kawamoto and, 152; for Minamata disease, 12, 143–50; versus money, 145, 154

rights, 119

right-wing politics, 67–69

rocks, on reclaimed land, 121–24, 136, 149*f*, 184

sabani, 123

sacred places, 122–24, 181–82

Sanrizuka, 84

sardines, 26, 33

Sashiki, 37

sashimi, 37

Sato Eisaku, 57

sayori, 33

Schindler's List, 132

school, 49–51, 53–55, 77; on Minamata disease, 12, 54–55; sports day, 37; and traditions, 170–71

sea cucumber, 33

sea urchins, 33

Self-Defense Forces, 68–69

shellfish, 33

shien, 184

Shimizu Self-Defense Force base, 68–69

Shimojima, 25

Shinagawa, 141

Shiranui Sea, 23*f*, 26; coast, population of, 3–4; fish from, 166–67; map, x

Shiranui Sea Fishermen's Union, 74

shirogo, 33

shizen, 165

Showa Denko, 8, 133–34

sin, Ogata on, 122, 146

Smith, W. Eugene, 9

socialism, 57, 76, 153

soil erosion, 166

Soshisha Minamata Disease Center, 10, 82–83, 88; Ogata on, 16n45

spirits, 141; of boat, 37; transmission of, 156. *See also* gods; religion spiritual community, 170, 172; Oiwa on, 185

spiritual quest, nervous breakdown as, 184–85

"A Statement of Original Vow," 121–22

stewardship, Ogata on, 121

St. Lawrence Corporation, 13–14

stones, on reclaimed land, 121–24, 136, 149f, 184

striped mullet, 33

students, and Minamata movement, 9, 75–76

suffering: Buddha and, 154; of Ogata Fukumatsu, 40–41, 44–45, 49

Sugimoto Eiko, 18, 21n1

Sugimoto Yu, 18

Sugimura Kunio, 80–81

sustainable development, 133

Suwa Festival, 37

Suzuki, David, 182–83

sweet pomelo, 33

Sympathy Agreement, 7, 58, 143

System: and Minamata movement, 88, 93, 145; Ogata on, 97, 155–56, 178

tachiuo, 26, 167, 167f, 179

tai, 26, 74, 166

takarago, 162

Tanaka (gangster), 63–65, 67–70; family of, 64; girlfriend of, 63–64

Tanaka Ayako, 5–6

Tanaka Jitsuko, 5–6

Tanaka Shizuko, 5–6

Tanaka Shozo, 184

Tani Yoichi, 101

technology: in fishing, 35; Ogata on, 13, 97, 173

television, Ogata on, 97, 178

tides, 35, 44, 165

Todd, Loretta, 183–84

Tokoyo, 14, 19f, 23f, 35, 106, 107f; building of, 103–8; first voyage of, 109–10; launching of, 17–21; meaning of name, 105

Tokyo, voyage to, 136–41

traditional peoples, 156–57; in Canada, 183–84; Ogata on, 178; wisdom of, 167–69

trawl netting, 26

trees, 34, 136, 166; cutting, ceremony for, 73

Tsubodan, 5

Tsuchimoto Noriaki, 97, 141

turtles, 165

typhoons, 129, 140

urami, 83f

utasebune, 136–41, 139f

villagers, 25–27; and activism, 87–88; and compensation payments, 148, 150; and festivals, 37, 51–52, 169–70; and Masato's return, 73; meetings of, 31; and Minamata disease, 5–6, 21n1, 58–59; resistance by, 171–72; rivalries of, 52, 55; and students, 75–76; traditions of, 167–70, 169f

Wakashio, 73–77

walking, 134–35

weddings, 37

Westernization, Ogata on, 153

women: and festivals, 169–70; and fishing, 33; and rhythms, 165

wooden boats, 17, 104–5, 123

World War II: and fishing industry, 26; legacy of, dealing with, 129–34

yakuza, 63–65, 67, 70, 82

Yanagida Koichi, 95; meaning of name, 97

Yokkaichi asthma pulmonary diseases, 10

Yoshii Masazumi, 12

Yunoura fisherman's union, protests by, 75f

Yuuan, 23f, 175, 178

Yuuantei Ooutsuke, 175. *See also* Ogata Masato

About . . .

THE AUTHOR

Oiwa Keibo (also known as Tsuji Shin'ichi) is an anthropologist and environmental activist teaching at Meiji Gakuin University in Yokohama. He founded the conservation organization, Sloth Club, to protect sloths and their habitat in Ecuador and to promote a more conscious way of living. His publications include the book *Slow Is Beautiful*.

THE NARRATOR

Ogata Masato is a fisherman and activist in Kumamoto, Japan.

THE TRANSLATOR

Karen Colligan-Taylor is professor emerita of Japanese Studies at the University of Alaska–Fairbanks. Her translations include *Sandakan Brothel No. 8: An Episode in the History of Lower-class Japanese Women* by Yamazaki Tomoko.

Asian Voices
Series Editor: Mark Selden

Identity in Okinawa
by Matthew Allen

Woman, Man, Bangkok: Sex, Love, and Popular Culture in Thailand
by Scot Barmé

Tales of Tibet: Sky Burials, Prayer Wheels, and Wind Horses
edited and translated by Herbert Batt, foreword by Tsering Shakya

Comfort Woman: A Filipina's Story of Prostitution and Slavery under the Japanese Military
by Maria Rosa Henson, introduction by Yuki Tanaka

Japan's Past, Japan's Future: One Historian's Odyssey
by Ienaga Saburō, translated and introduced by Richard H. Minear

Growing Up Untouchable in India: A Dalit Autobiography
by Vasant Moon, translated by Gail Omvedt, introduction by Eleanor Zelliot

Red Is Not the Only Color: Contemporary Chinese Fiction on Love and Sex between Women, Collected Stories
edited by Patricia Sieber

Unbroken Spirits: Nineteen Years in South Korea's Gulag
by Suh Sung, translated by Jean Inglis, foreword by James Palais

Bitter Flowers, Sweet Flowers: East Timor, Indonesia, and the World Community
edited by Richard Tanter, Mark Selden, and Stephen R. Shalom

Voicing Concerns: Contemporary Chinese Critical Inquiry
edited by Gloria Davies, conclusion by Geremie Barmé

Dear General MacArthur: Letters from the Japanese during the American Occupation
by Sodei Rinjirō, edited by John Junkerman, foreword by John W. Dower